Fix My Shoulder

Fix My Shoulder

A Guide to Preventing and Healing from Injury and Strain

George Demirakos

ROWMAN & LITTLEFIELD
Lanham • Boulder • New York • London

Published by Rowman & Littlefield
A wholly owned subsidary of The Rowman & Littlefield Publishing Group, Inc.
4501 Forbes Boulevard, Suite 200, Lanham, Maryland 20706
www.rowman.com

Unit A, Whitacre Mews, 26-34 Stannary Street, London SE11 4AB

British Library Cataloguing in Publication Information Available

Library of Congress Cataloging-in-Publication Data

The hardback edition of this book was previously cataloged by the Library of
Congress as follows:

Demirakos, George.
  Fix my shoulder : a guide to preventing and healing from injury and strain /
George Demirakos.
      pages cm
  Includes bibliographical references and index.
  1. Shoulder—Wounds and injuries—Prevention—Popular works.
2. Shoulder—Wounds and injuries—Treatment—Popular works.   3. Shoulder—
Anatomy—Popular works.   I. Title.
  RD557.5.D44 2014
  617.5'72044—dc23
                                                        2014017194

ISBN 978-1-4422-3337-9 (cloth : alk. paper)
ISBN 978-1-4422-7585-0 (pbk. : alk. paper)
ISBN 978-1-4422-3338-6 (electronic)

Printed in the United States of America

Contents

Disclaimer   vii

Acknowledgments   ix

Introduction   xi

Chapter 1:   The Nuts and Bolts of the Shoulder   1

Chapter 2:   Of Rotator Cuffs, Injuries, and Words Ending in——*itis*   11

Chapter 3:   The Pain   37

Chapter 4:   The Fix   59

Chapter 5:   Fix Your Posture, Too   87

Chapter 6:   For Workout Warriors, Moves to Avoid—Or at Least Modify   111

Chapter 7:   Your Super Shoulder   123

Notes   151

Bibliography   155

Index   159

Contents

Disclaimer

This book represents reference material only. It is not intended as a medical manual, and the data presented here are meant to assist the reader in making informed choices regarding wellness. This book is not a replacement for treatment(s) that the reader's personal physician may have suggested. If the reader believes he or she is experiencing a medical issue, professional medical help is recommended. Mention of particular products, companies, or authorities in this book does not entail endorsement by the publisher or author.

First speak to your doctor before beginning any exercise program.

Even a minor rotator cuff injury, unevaluated and untreated, can lead to decreasing or eliminating the normal function of your shoulder. Don't wait. Make that appointment today!

Acknowledgments

I am deeply grateful and appreciative of all the people who have helped me bring this initial dream into actual fruition. I could not have done this alone without so many people knowingly and unknowingly guiding me and cheering me on to make this book. To all of you out there, thank you so much.

To Sarah Jane Freymann, my amazing agent, who believed in me when no one else would and who took a chance. I would not be here if not due to you.

To Susanne Margolis, my magician, who waves her magic wand and turns some dry, medical reading into a joyous fun story that people would want to read.

To my publishing company, Rowman and Littlefield, and to my editor, Suzanne Stasiak-Silva. With her confident and calming personality, she would instantly take my stress away and make my progress into this writing world so much easier.

I also want to thank Kathryn Knigge, Laura Reiter, Flannery Scott, and everyone at Rowman and Littlefield for the amazing work that they did with my pictures in the book. Thanks, guys!

To my parents, who encouraged me to follow my dreams and never stop trying with a smile on my face, as well as my sisters, who have inspired me to give as much as I can to others as they have given back to me.

To all the people out there who gave me strength to go ahead and write this book, inspiring me to become the best therapist I can be and keep cheering for me all the way. I would personally like to thank the following amazing therapists: Bahram Jam, David Campbell, Joel Cyr, Julie Gardner, Karen Litzy, Ann McMillan, and Frederic Watine. If you have ever been treated by them, consider yourselves very lucky.

To the countless other therapists who I have met and who have enriched my practice with their golden nuggets of knowledge and skill—all the physiotherapists, athletic therapists, osteopaths, chiropractors, and doctors. Thank you so much.

Special thanks also goes to the following people without whose encouragement and goodwill help, this book would still be a dream of mine: Robert Soroka, Lynn Betts, Roger Casgrain, and Alain April.

I would also like to take this opportunity to thank my spiritual motivators, Mr. Arnold Schwarzenegger, Dr. Mehmet Oz, Miss Jillian Michaels, and Mr. Gordon Ramsay. I have never met them, but through their hard work and undeniable determination, they helped me believe in myself and overcome obstacles that I didn't think I could. To them, I say thanks.

I would also like to thank Augustus Mantelis from Augustus Photography and his crew for the beautiful pictures taken. A special thank you goes out to Mindy Shear Poupko from Mindy Shear Cosmetics for making us look young and amazing.

A special shout out goes to the models, Kendra Toothill, Talia Erdan, and Martin Durand, who came in to help at the last minute, and did a fantastic job. I am very lucky to call them my friends.

I would also like to thank all my patients who I have had the pleasure of meeting and treating their shoulder problems over the years. I hope that this book helps you find the relief that you are looking for.

I would like to thank my son and daughter who put up with the fact that daddy had to work and could not play with them everyday. You are the best and I love you so much.

And lastly, none of these ideas could have happened if it were not for my shining light in my life, my wife, Frankie. She has been through thick and thin, all the ups and downs, and her beautiful smile always made me do things that I thought I could never do. She is the reason why you are reading this book. You are my life, my everything. Thank you for being my best friend.

Introduction

It was a deep-rooted habit of long standing: Every time Lisa got into her car, she automatically tossed her bag into the back seat, knowing that if she needed anything from it—her wallet, her glasses, a pack of tissues— she could easily reach around the seat back and haul the bag up front. So today when she needed change for a bridge toll, she reached back as always, grabbed the bag handle, started to raise the bag from the back seat, and—wow!—felt a pain so searing she almost lost control of the car. By the time Lisa was able to pull over to try to massage the pain away, she could barely move her shoulder at all.

Matt is twenty-eight, a lawyer, and a self-confessed "gym rat." Because he's never sure how long his work day will be, he tries to hit the gym early every morning: a little cardio followed by some serious weight training, his main focus. Curls, crunches, presses, lifts, pull-downs, pushdowns: In pursuit of washboard abs—which look great!—Matt does it all. And despite the fact that he's been doing it for a while, he recently made the classic training mistake: too much weight too soon and insufficient rest between sets. He felt it right away—stabs of fiery pain in his shoulder.

Matt knew enough to ice the pain, and he prudently stayed away from the gym for a few days. But he must have come back too soon, because the instant he tried a set of shoulder presses, he was stopped cold by overpowering pain. Forget the buff body and the ability to bench-press 250; Matt was out of commission.

A colleague of Matt's, Andrew, eschews the gym workouts but is a passionate weekend sportsman who can easily play two tennis matches on Saturday and be ready for a round of golf on Sunday. He was familiar with the terms *tennis elbow*, *tennis knee*, and *tennis toe* but had never heard of *tennis shoulder* till he woke up with the pain of it one night. On the court the next Saturday, Andrew found he could barely raise his serving arm at all, much less fire off an ace. And when he approached the tee for Sunday's round of golf, he had no power in his right arm at all; he felt like he was trying to swing the club with his left arm—and it just couldn't be done.

Then there's Tyler, the options trader who sits at a desk in front of four computer monitors from the moment the market opens in the morning till the moment it closes in the afternoon—with no break. For those six-and-a-half stationary hours, Tyler is scrunched over with his head leaning forward into the monitors as if he could will the numbers to go his way. His shoulder blades are stretched apart so he can turn his arms inward and keep his hands at the ready to hit the keyboard in a split nanosecond, which, in Tyler's view, is all the time he has to respond to any market shifts.

Last week, when Tyler went in for his annual physical, he told his doctor he thought the stress of the trading job was getting to him: he was feeling it in his shoulder, which was killing him.

Does any of this sound familiar? Sure it does. It's shoulder pain—the surprise twinge of pain when, like Lisa, you reach around behind you, maybe for something as simple as tucking in your shirt or blouse. Or, like Andrew, your face tightens into a wince when you stretch up to take something down from an upper shelf—a sharp ache followed by the sense that your whole arm has gone weak. Maybe you know the misery of lying awake at night because of shoulder pain that makes it hurt to turn over. You just can't get comfortable no matter which side you lie on or what position you twist yourself into.

Maybe you work in an office and find that you're always rubbing the back of your neck or shrugging your shoulders or having to get up from your desk chair and walk around for a few minutes. Or perhaps your work requires manual labor and the use of your arms to lift, haul, and carry—if you're a firefighter perhaps, or a construction worker, or work in a factory or warehouse—and you've begun to feel you're losing the muscle power you always relied upon. Worst of all, maybe you're a parent who finds you have to check yourself before you pick up the baby; you're just not sure you feel the strength you used to feel.

Its shoulder pain, and it's slowing you down, limiting your movement, affecting your life.

The shoulder is the most mobile joint in the body. It enjoys an amazing range of motion; it can rotate 360 degrees and can extend upward, sideways, across the body, outward, inward—every which way. That makes it the most useful joint we have, and, not surprisingly, we use it the most. Lifting, pushing, pulling, throwing, catching, hugging: the shoulder experiences more motion than any other joint. So it is perhaps not surprising that, sooner or later, it becomes overtaxed—fatigued. After all, as with anything, if you keep applying the same pressure over and over, the strength and stability of the structure being pressured will wear down. That's what happens to the shoulder, and when it does, it's not only painful; it can also stop you in your tracks, limiting your ability to do even simple things you're used to doing.

When we injure the shoulder in some way, it naturally stops working as it should. It won't rotate the full 360 degrees or lift quite as high or pull quite as forcefully. That makes it hard to pick something up from the floor or pull something down from overhead. Spending hours in front of the computer becomes torture, as it was for Tyler. Lifting groceries out of the car and carrying them into the house becomes an ordeal. Weekend warriors can no longer enjoy the activities they once prized—just ask Andrew. New grandparents can't reach out comfortably to hold the baby.

And the hard truth is that the wearing down that life in general does to our shoulders will probably only grow worse as we grow older. Our bodies tend to lose muscle and bone mass as we age, and we become more susceptible to the aches and pains that may result.

But neither the weakness nor the pain is inevitable. The shoulder can be fixed, and the pain can go away. First, there's a fix that cures the weakness and ends the pain. But there's also a fix that can serve as a preventive, so that you never have to lose the strength, stability, and range of motion of the shoulder at all. I can show you both, and that is what I am going to do in this book.

THE KEY PROBLEM—AND THE KEY TO FIXING IT

There can be any number of triggering causes for shoulder trouble—a wrong or awkward movement, overuse, bad posture—and there is a range of results of shoulder injury, each with its own name. Lisa's injury resulted in frozen shoulder—officially, adhesive capsulitis; Matt's rush to get back to his workout exacerbated what we would probably call *bursitis*; Andrew's dead-arm syndrome was likely the result of shoulder instability or imbalance; and Tyler suffered all the aches and discomfort of tendinitis. But whatever the name, the bottom line is that it is all about the rotator cuff, which is why it's essential to understand precisely what that means.

There's also another key to the problem, made particularly vivid to me in working with my professional-athlete patients who play for the Montreal Canadiens of the National Hockey League or for the Canadian Tennis Championships. It's all about the supporting muscles—a whole group of them that underpin and assist the work of the rotator cuff even though they are, in a sense, nowhere near it. Their job, however, is to support the supporters and stabilize the stabilizers, and what is now abundantly clear and confirmed by research is that you need to strengthen these muscles too. They may not be the star players in the shoulder's flexibility, but their supporting role as strengtheners of the strengtheners makes them equally important in fixing your shoulder. In the pages that follow, you'll learn to pay these muscles the attention they deserve, and in doing so, you'll find a therapeutic fix for your shoulder pain that is more than the sum of the parts.

This book was written in order to empower and educate people on the causes of shoulder pain, looking primarily at the rotator cuff, and surrounding muscles. It is a goal of mine for people to understand how and why they got shoulder problems, and how to get better. It all starts with a game plan. This book has also been written to help answer questions that people really want to ask their doctor or allied health professional, but do not. It might be that they forgot to ask or are shy and embarrassed to ask their doctor.

While this book in no way takes the place of medical advice, having a deeper understanding of what is really going on in your shoulder will allow you to have an informed conversation with your doctor, so that you can both come up with a proper game plan for getting you better. I believe that no matter what sex or race you are, what language you speak, and where you live in the world, if you are in shoulder pain, this book can help. It might not fix your problem completely but it will at least steer you in the right direction.

Most people might experience some kind of nagging shoulder discomfort or pain at some point in their lives. Some of these aches and pains might get resolved naturally, and we never have to think about them again. Some shoulder issues might not get resolved that quickly, and some of you might have shoulder issues that have lasted for a long time and you can't get rid of the pain. I hope that I can shed some light on this.

As you'll learn in greater detail in chapters 1 and 2, the rotator cuff is actually four muscles—and their tendons—that stabilize the shoulder joint. Unlike the hip joint's ball-and-socket structure, the shoulder joint has only a shallow groove. That shallowness is what gives the shoulder its free-swinging range of motion, but it takes four rotator cuff muscles working together, along with some supporting muscles, to keep it stable.

That means that any sort of weakness in the rotator cuff is the starting point of shoulder troubles. Fixing the shoulder is therefore first and foremost about strengthening the muscles of the rotator cuff. Ditto for preventing shoulder troubles in the first place.

The way the shoulder works with respect to the rest of the body and that it doesn't move just by itself is very interesting. For example, if your rib cage and neck are stiff and you are hunched over, you might not be able to lift your shoulder all the way up or as far as you would like. We then go through some definitions to give you that information that you might have been thinking about—for example, what does the word *tendonitis* really mean?

Chapter 3 will go into an area that I get a lot of questions about: pain. I will also touch on the debate between the age-old question: what should I put on my shoulder: ice or heat?

Chapter 4 represents the heart of the book, called *The Fix*. Here is where I explain the different type of exercises that you can do, how many and how often, and what to watch out for. You will get different range-of-motion and strength routines, starting from the easy and progressively getting more advanced. These routines will guide you to slowly develop your shoulder's full flexibility and strengthen your shoulder in every direction to make you feel good and confident with performing everyday tasks. For those weekend warriors out there who want to get stronger at throwing a football around or going for a swim, these routines will enable you to enjoy your sport again.

We changed gears a bit with chapter 5, with talk on posture. I am sure we have all heard from our moms to "sit up straight" and while we all have good intentions, we don't really keep the posture we really want—from sitting at the office to home life. We will speak of some posture "do and don'ts," as well as how to make yourself the posture envy of your office.

Next, in chapter 6, we will go through exercises or movements that you should avoid if you are experiencing an injured shoulder. Some of the exercises chosen may surprise you. If done incorrectly, some of your favorite exercises done in the gym may actually be hurting your shoulder, causing unnecessary pain and suffering. We will go through what you can do about it in a safe and effective way.

In the last chapter, chapter 7, called *Your Super Shoulder*, I will give you some shoulder exercises that might be familiar to you and other exercises that might not be well-known. These exercises are normally introduced by highly skilled professional trainers and therapists to their patients, but I have found them to be the very best exercises out there. We will also create some exercise routines to get you nice and ready for some of your favorite sports.

Although this book has been written to be read from the beginning to the end first, I would also suggest and encourage you to use the book as a reference, reading the parts that really pertain to you. Bring this book, if you like, to your doctor; by using the information here, you can really help speed up your understanding and make your game plan that much easier.

I truly hope that you find this book entertaining and informative. I really wrote it to help as many people out there as possible who have shoulder problems and want answers to their questions. I am a physiotherapist by occupation and I love my job. I love helping people, and I hope, in some way, this book will help your shoulder pain find relief and improve your quality of life.

WHO AM I?

I am a licensed physical therapist and certified athletic trainer who has worked with an NHL hockey team, the Canadian Tennis Championships, and with athletes in the 2012 Olympic Games. I am currently the clinic director, senior physiotherapist, and leader of the sports medicine team of the Club Sportif MAA in downtown Montreal, and have served on the Associate Boards of the McGill Faculty of Physiotherapy, and Sports Physiotherapy Canada—Canada's professional association for sports physiotherapists. I recently worked as the physiotherapist on the set of *X-Men: Days of Future Past.*

I hope you enjoy the book as much as I did writing it.

1

The Nuts and Bolts of the Shoulder

"As for me, all I know is that I know nothing."

—Socrates

Knowing *something* about the shoulder is the right place to start. After all, the shoulder is a joint we very rarely think about unless and until the persistent twinge or repeated limitation makes us sit up and take notice. Once we understand just what this joint is and does, and once we see how it works, we gain an appreciation of all that is involved in keeping the shoulder operational and at its best.

The shoulder is an amazing mechanism, one of the great "inventions" of human evolution. It offers the greatest range of motion of any part of the body, enabling a range of functions so essential we simply don't think about them. We don't think about lifting the arm to reach for something, about pushing an object along a table top, about pulling something toward us, about tossing a ball—or pitching one hard—about catching the ball that's been tossed or pitched to us, about wrapping someone we love in a hug. Yet it's the shoulder that makes all those actions possible.

To accommodate the variety of those movements, however, the shoulder gives up some strength and stability. This is why shoulders get injured, and it's why you feel the pain of those injuries. It all has to do with the way the shoulder works—how the bones, joints, and numerous muscles that make up the shoulder function together. It is why they sometimes don't function together all that effectively or without causing you the twinges and aches—and outright shrieks of pain—that can so limit your life. Shoulders can weaken and can be destabilized, and that's where the trouble starts.

THE BONES OF THE SHOULDER

The bones of the shoulder are the clavicle, the scapula, and the humerus.

The clavicle, or collarbone, is a long bone that connects your arm—that is, your upper limb—to the rest of your body. You know it as that bulging bone on your chest that you can easily touch. Connected to the scapula, the clavicle is also an attachment point for muscles and ligaments. It is little wonder it got its name—*clavicula* is Latin for "little key"—because it rotates along its axis like a key when you lift your arm out to the side, a process known as *abduction*.

The scapula, or shoulder blade, is basically a triangular bone on which the famous rotator cuff muscles lie. The ball-like head of the humerus fits into a depression in the scapula called the *glenoid fossa*, and the scapula thus connects the humerus to the clavicle. The scapula also boasts a bony summit, called the *acromion process*, which forms the highest point of the shoulder. The name "scapula" is said to come from a Greek word, *scaptein*, which, I can assure you, means to dig; the ancients thought of it as a small shovel.

Finally, the humerus is the largest bone of the upper arm. It connects to the rest of the body through the scapula. Since it is one of the longest bones in the body, it is also one of the most commonly fractured. Many muscles end at the humerus—at places called *insertions*—and many others start there, at places called *origins*. A big bumpy structure on top of the humerus, called the *greater tubercle*, is where most of the rotator cuff muscles connect.

What holds these three bones together? Various joints in the shoulder.

JOINTS OF THE SHOULDER

What is a joint anyhow? It is simply a point where two or more bones come together. What joints do is allow the bones to move in different directions, and the body is filled with all shapes and sizes of joints.

There are four major joints in the shoulder:

The glenohumeral (G/H) joint,
The acromioclavicular (A/C) joint,
The sternoclavicular (S/C) joint, and
The scapulothoracic (S/T) joint.

Let's take them one at a time.

The glenohumeral, or G/H joint, is the one we primarily talk about when we speak of the shoulder joint. It comprises two distinct parts: the head of the humerus bone, and the glenoid fossa groove in the scapula. That meeting point creates the glenohumeral joint. It is a simple ball-and-socket type of joint, similar to the mechanism of the hip. But there is a difference. The groove or fossa of the scapula, where the head of the humerus fits, is very shallow, in contrast to the deep groove of the hip socket.

It is that shallow scapular groove that gives the G/H joint its ample freedom but that is also a liability in terms of stability. That is, the G/H joint can fairly easily slip out of place. Say you trip and reach out an arm to break your fall as you hit the ground. That's a good way to dislocate your glenohumeral joint, especially if the muscles around the area are not strong enough. Therefore, the glenohumeral joint depends on the muscles around it more than on the bony structures or ligaments for its stability.[1]

But just consider all the movements the G/H joint lets you do. You can lift your arm in front of you—that's called *flexion*; extend your arm out behind you—*extension*; lift your arm to either side—*abduction*; stretch your arm across your body—*adduction*; turn your arm outward—*external rotation*; and turn your arm inward—*internal rotation*.

Normally, when you hear about somebody having a rotator cuff injury, it means that the back, or posterior, of the G/H joint has stiffened up, pushing all the other structures of the shoulder joint forward. When that happens, the shoulder can't go through its proper movements, so it tries to move by using the other joints, which eventually damages the area, causes pain, and of course impinges on the front or anterior part of your shoulder.

Loosening up the posterior part of the G/H joint will take some of the stress off the shoulder, which will greatly help with the healing. But it's important to remember that when it comes to stability, the G/H joint depends more on the muscles around it—namely, the rotator cuff muscles—than on the bones or ligaments.

The acromioclavicular joint, routinely called the A/C joint, is between your clavicle and the acromion or topmost part of your scapula. The A/C joint connects the shoulder to the rest of your body but is also important in holding the bones together as the arm goes through its full range of motion. The A/C joint sits above the rotator cuff. It can also become dislocated; such a dislocation is called a *separated shoulder*.

The sternoclavicular, or S/C joint, connects the clavicle to the breast bone, or sternum, in the front of your chest. This is a very stable joint. Because it barely moves, it is rarely injured, although injury is not impossible. The S/C joint is the only true connection between the shoulder and the chest cavity.

The scapulothoracic, or S/T joint, is not a true joint at all. It is actually a sliding "joint" located between the inner border of the scapula and the ribs numbered two through seven. Its job is to let the scapula move on the rib cage.[2] There are not actually any ligaments in the S/C joint, but certain muscles of the scapula move it smoothly up and down and in rotation with shoulder movement.

What holds this amazing mechanism in place and keeps it stable and soundly positioned? That's the job of tendons, ligaments, and capsules.

TENDONS, LIGAMENTS, CAPSULES

A tendon is a tough, dense band of connective tissue that is the natural continuation of a muscle; think of it as the endpoint of a muscle joined to a bone. Muscle is normally soft and pliable, but a tendon is like a cord. Rub your shoulder area and see if you come across something that feels like a cord; you're probably touching a tendon. Tendons are inelastic and made to withstand any tension placed on them. That's good, because tendons are responsible for helping the muscles contract. Along with muscles, tendons are designed to move bones around. Thanks to the bursa, a flat, fluid-filled sac located over a bone, tendons are able more or less to just glide smoothly and without resistance as they move—until they don't, of course, and that's what we call *bursitis*.

A ligament, on the other hand, is a structure made up of fibrous connective tissue, primarily long collagen fibers that connects one bone to another to form a joint. A ligament cannot, however, contract. When placed under tension, ligaments normally lengthen, whereas tendons do not.

A third positioning and stabilizing structure in the shoulder is called the *capsule*. It is really a sheathlike covering or envelope made up of ligaments that surround a joint. Three major ligaments surround the glenohumeral joint—the upper, middle, and lower glenohumeral ligaments—and they make up most of the capsule. It is in this capsule that the head of the humerus reaches the socket of the scapula.

What holds these structures together while at the same time enabling the shoulder to move through its extraordinary range of motion and of function is the set of muscles known as the *rotator cuff*.

ROTATOR CUFF MUSCLES

Four muscles make up the rotator cuff region; I call them the "fab four":

The supraspinatus muscle,
The infraspinatus muscle,
The teres minor muscle, and
The subscapularis muscle.

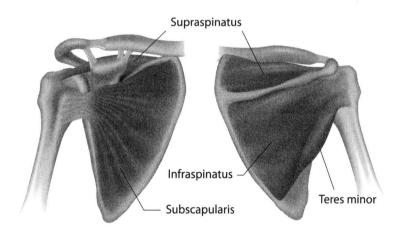

Muscles of the rotator cuff. *Alila Medical Media/Shutterstock*

The supraspinatus is perhaps the best known of these, mostly because it is the muscle that most commonly becomes torn or gets tendinitis. It is found at the upper part of the scapula, specifically in the back of the shoulder blade. Along with the deltoid muscle, it helps in abduction, moving the upper arm away from the body. It also helps stabilize the head of the humerus so that it doesn't move upward in the groove of the scapula.

A well-known study[3] found a significantly high level of electrical activity in the supraspinatus muscle tissue during the external rotation of the shoulder—that is, when you stretch your arm outward to the side. The study concluded therefore that the supraspinatus muscle can be trained through resisted external rotation of the shoulder—that is, by the use of weights—to turn the shoulder outward as well as inward.[4] It means that although officially your supraspinatus muscle is there to help extend your arm out to the side of your body, it can also work in external rotation.

The infraspinatus and teres minor muscles are located at the back of the shoulder blade and below the supraspinatus. These really small muscles are primarily responsible for external rotation. They also help prevent excessive backward and upward movement of the head of the humerus on the scapula. This holds the humeral head in the glenoid fossa during movements of the shoulder joint, which in turn works in a profound way to stabilize the G/H joint.

The subscapularis muscle, the biggest and strongest of the fab four rotator cuff muscles, takes up the entire front part of the shoulder blade, which faces the ribs. Its most important job is to help turn the shoulder toward the body—internal rotation—and to adduct the arm, or stretch it across the body. It helps stabilize the humerus, keeping it from moving forward and upward.

If these rotator cuff muscles are not strong enough to hold everything together, problems arise—tendinitis, for example—and the shoulder may be impinged anteriorly or in the front. Although each rotator cuff muscle controls a different individual shoulder movement, all of the fab four work together to stabilize your shoulder. In that sense, they really are not separate muscles. Rather, they are four flat tendons fused together to form a cuff that surrounds the humerus—just the way a blood pressure (BP) cuff surrounds your arm when your doctor measures your BP. It has in fact been determined that the rotator cuff muscles all contract and stabilize your shoulder when you start moving your arm to do something.[5] So as you can appreciate, any weakness or imbalance in this area can start the process toward impingement and those pesky problems—shoulder pain, shoulder weakness, loss of shoulder function—that you want to get rid of and stay free from forever.

That is why strengthening the rotator cuff is so extremely important.

SCAPULAR STABILIZING MUSCLES

There are other stabilizing muscles that are almost equally important for the health of the shoulder. Among them are:

Rhomboids
Lower Trapezius
Serratus Anterior

Rhomboids are the two diamond-shaped muscles that start at the side of your upper spine and connect to the inner or medial part of your shoulder blades. One of these is called the *rhomboid major*, the other the *rhomboid minor*, and as you'd guess, the rhomboid major is bigger. In fact, it is twice the size of the minor. But both muscles do the same thing—namely, they bring your shoulder blades together, and they lift and downward-rotate your scapula, as does your levator scapula, the skeletal muscle at the back and side of your neck that we all tend to start massaging when we feel tired or tense—or both.

Many office workers who tend to slouch in their chairs in front of the computer typically suffer from weakened rhomboids, and there's a simple way to tell. The clue is shoulder blades that "stick out" on a person in a standing position; that's a pretty clear indication of rhomboids that are so weak they are unable to keep the shoulder blade flat against the rib cage. It is a weakness that can definitely contribute to shoulder pain.

You know where your "trap" or trapezius muscles are. Like everyone else, you're always trying to rub your traps—at least, your upper traps— press on them, or do something to loosen them up. But again, those are the upper trapezius muscles between your ear and your shoulder, and in fact, the uppers are not the traps you should be worrying about.

Like the rhomboids, the trapezius muscle is the shape of a diamond, with upper traps and lower traps corresponding to the two halves of the diamond. The lower traps start at the bottom of the thoracic vertebrae on your rib cage and connect to the shoulder blade. It is the job of the upper traps to lift the shoulder blade as well as rotate it upward, while the lower traps pull the shoulder blade down and rotate it upward. (There are also middle traps that bring the shoulder blades together to the spine, just like the rhomboids.)

When your shoulders start to droop—as, for example, when you are sitting at your desk—the upper traps will pull your shoulder blades up to your ears, giving you those awful knots or spasms in your neck. This happens because your upper traps are probably stronger than your lower traps and are winning the tug of war. If your lower traps are strengthened enough to counterbalance the upper ones, they will pull the shoulder blades back down, thus lowering your chances of experiencing spasms and pain. That's why the lower traps deserve a great deal of your attention.

The serratus anterior is a muscle that is different from the rest. Shaped like a saw, the serratus anterior starts at the front of the rib cage and finishes at the shoulder blade in the back. Its main goal is to keep and hold the shoulder blade against the rib cage in the back where it winds around to the back. It can also bring the shoulder blade forward, which is why it is commonly called "the boxer's muscle," the one that goes into action when a boxer throws a punch. But what is particularly interesting about this muscle is its relation to the shoulder blade. It is the most powerful upward rotator of the scapula and will tilt the scapula backward, keeping it in its rightful place, stabilized against the rib cage to counter the reactive forces of the free limb. That's doubly good because in so doing, the serratus anterior neutralizes its counterpart muscle, the pectoralis minor.

The Pectoralis Minor and the Biceps

The pectoralis minor muscle starts on your ribs and ends up connecting to your scapula. Although the pec minor performs numerous helpful functions in the body, it tends to tighten if you sit slouched for too long. (You're not slouching *now*, are you?) When that happens, it tilts the scapula forward and rotates it downward. This then decreases the possible range of motion of your shoulder, specifically affecting your ability to lift your arm up. Obviously, therefore, if you can strengthen your serratus anterior, it will come to your rescue and balance you out.

Most people don't realize that the biceps muscle—official name: biceps brachii—is also involved with rotator cuff injuries. The "bi" in *biceps* means that the muscle is really in two parts, one long and one short, both of which attach to the radius bone in the forearm. The long head of the biceps, also the larger of the two parts of this muscle, goes into the deep part of the shoulder joint itself anteriorly, right at the front end of the humerus bone. This is an area of the shoulder in which you can typically experience pain or discomfort. For example, if you feel pain or discomfort when you stand up after sitting at your desk for a while, it's very likely that the long head of your biceps has been affected, especially if you haven't used your arm for a while.

The short head of the biceps connects into the projecting part of the shoulder blade and rarely gets injured.

Now as everyone knows, the biceps bend the elbow and turn the wrist outward; the latter is called *supination*. But what you might not know is that the long head of the biceps is also involved in overhead lifting movements, both when you bend your arm and when you rotate it externally or turn outward. That's why the biceps can also be involved in shoulder injury.

Pectoralis Major, Latissimus Dorsi, Teres Major

Everybody has heard of your pecs and lats muscles. Pecs are the pectoralis muscles of the chest, including the pec minor we just talked about. Lats are the latissimus dorsi in your back, starting from just underneath your armpits to your lower back.

The teres major muscle is a smaller muscle located near the region of the shoulder where the rest of your rotator cuff muscles are located.

These three muscles perform several major functions for controlling arm movements, but the main reason they're in a book about shoulder pain is that all three internally rotate the shoulder. Why is that important?

The rotator cuff muscles that externally rotate your shoulder are much smaller than the internal rotators. If your rotator cuff muscles are weak, that creates a muscle imbalance. When the internal muscles are stronger than your external muscles, moving your shoulder to perform certain tasks can throw your shoulder biomechanics "out of whack" and cause pain and stiffness. That is why it is so important to strengthen the external rotators of your shoulders.

In a recent study, researchers found that a forward-tipping scapula and weak serratus anterior muscle were directly related to shoulder impingement problems from overhead movement.[6]

What is the bottom line of all this? It isn't just the famous rotator cuff muscles that need strengthening if you're going to fix that shoulder. You'll also need to strengthen a number of other muscles—supporting players that nevertheless perform essential roles in a healthy shoulder.

CHAPTER ONE SUMMARY

- The three major bones of the shoulder are the scapula or shoulder blade, humerus or arm bone, and clavicle or collarbone.
- The four major joints of the shoulder are the glenohumeral or G/H joint, acromioclavicular or A/C joint, sternoclavicular or S/C joint, and the scapulothoracic or S/T joint.
- The four main muscles of the rotator cuff are: the supraspinatus, infraspinatus, teres minor, and subscapularis.
- The main job of the supraspinatus is to lift the arm away from the body—to abduct the arm.
- The main job of the infraspinatus and teres minor is to turn the arm away from the body—to rotate the arm externally.
- The main job of the subscapularis is to turn the arm in toward the body—to rotate the arm internally.
- Your external rotators are anatomically smaller than your internal rotators, so failure to strengthen the external rotators can result in muscle imbalances and pain.
- The rotator muscles contract and stabilize the shoulder before an activity with the arm is initiated.
- People who sit in a slouched position for long periods of time develop forward-tilting shoulders resulting from the tightening of the pec minor muscle and upper traps plus a weak serratus anterior and lower trap.

2

Of Rotator Cuffs, Injuries, and Words Ending in——*itis*

"I would rather entertain and hope that people learned something than educate people and hope they were entertained."

—Walt Disney

What does it really mean to have a shoulder injury or shoulder pain? The overall term for such problems is a *shoulder impingement syndrome*, but that's about as precise a description as *sciatica* or *shin splints*. People who swim a lot call their pain *swimmer's shoulder*, while people who play a lot of ball games call it *thrower's shoulder*. Whatever you call it, shoulder impingement syndrome is about pain that is in some way limiting the movement of the individual's shoulder. But what does it really mean?

Let us go through some important and fundamental terms and definitions below. Having a better understanding of the words themselves will give you a much clearer vision of what the doctor or the allied health practitioner is trying to explain to you.

TENDONITIS AND OTHER——*ITISES*

What's a Tendonitis?

Before we understand what a tendonitis is, we need to know the definition of what *itis* means. It is a suffix derived from the Greek language, meaning an inflammation of a structure. For example, tendonitis is an inflammation of a tendon. A capsulitis is an inflammation of a capsule, primarily being your G/H joint, but not necessarily in every case.

Normal

Rotator cuff problems

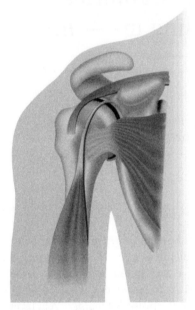
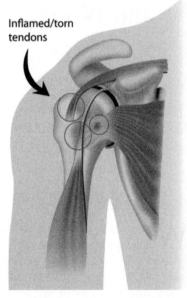

Inflamed/torn tendons

Rotator cuff and long head of biceps tendinitis. *Alila Medical Media/Shutterstock*

A bursitis is the inflammation of your bursa, which is a sac-like structure, cushioning and absorbing the pressure or stress placed between two structures, normally between a muscle and a bone. The shoulder contains eight different types of bursa—the most of any joint in the body.

Let's Talk a Bit About Pain

What is it really? Pain is described as a highly unpleasant physical sensation caused by illness or injury. Because describing how we perceive pain and our tolerance of pain is different from person to person, it is difficult to describe and to properly define it. Pain is a signal or sensation that comes from your nerves. Keeping in mind that pain is a signal to the brain that something is wrong, it is, in my opinion, to figure out what is causing the pain first, rather than just treating the pain.

Once you have seen the doctor, and other nonmusculoskeletal things have been ruled out (i.e., fractures, dislocations, or other medical conditions), and your condition has been classified as a tendonitis, or an impingement shoulder syndrome, it is then that therapists have to really look at two major things:

1. How is your range of motion (ROM) of your shoulder region and all the structures around it?
2. How is your shoulder's strength or lack of strength?

When someone has a properly diagnosed shoulder issue, just taking medications or just doing some exercises will not fix everything. I believe a combined approach (bringing down the inflammation with medication if necessary, icing the area, with ROM and strength exercises) will help your condition get better overall.

What is most important to me when I see a patient is what the deficiencies in their shoulder range of motion are and where their lack of strength is. This is the information I try to get when I see my patient in their initial evaluation. What's tight, weak, and strong in the area? My primary focus when I look at my patient is what is not working versus how it should be working. I work on those things first before I look at anything else.

Why Do We Get Tendonitis?

A minor, repetitive incorrect move done all the time, every day most likely causes a tendonitis. Anyone can get tendonitis, but it is most common between the ages of 20 and 40, when the tendon has been pulled more than it is accustomed to.

A rotator cuff tendonitis can come from a variety of things: from sport activities like throwing a baseball, serving a tennis ball, or swimming incorrectly, to everyday chores like lifting heavy groceries from the supermarket, raking leaves or gardening. A lot of individuals can get rotator cuff tendonitis from just typing with a poor posture position at their computer. Even athletes, whose job it is to train and to excel for their specific sport, get tendonitis all the time. Most of the time tendonitis is due to repetitive microtrauma due to continuous faulty movements.

Left undiagnosed and not treated properly and quickly, a tendinitis can turn into a tendinosis, which is a long-lasting tendinitis. Eventually, it can worsen, depending on the degree, into a chronic shoulder muscle tear or even something serious: a frozen shoulder.

Frozen Shoulder

Frozen shoulder, officially known as *adhesive capsulitis*, is normally defined by pain and loss of motion in the glenohumeral joint of the shoulder. It can cause the capsule surrounding the shoulder joint to contract and form a lot of scar tissue. This will cause the area to become stiff and inflamed creating a loss of range of motion and pain. The cause is not really understood and can greatly frustrate and confuse patients, as well as their caregivers, due to the long length of time needed to recover. It can last from a few months up to three years or more in some cases. Frozen shoulder is not just an orthopedic problem. Rather, like rheumatoid arthritis, it is a systemic condition and can be associated with individuals who are postmenopausal or have diabetes, alcoholism, or hyperthyroidism. It can also happen with immobilization due to surgery.

Let me be clear that frozen shoulder is not osteoarthritis. The literature seems to suggest that adhesive capsulitis might have an autoimmune component. This is when the body starts to attack healthy tissue in the capsule. It can happen after an injury or trauma to the shoulder region, but not necessarily in all cases. There would also be a lack of fluid that would make the movements even smaller and more restrictive. It happens to approximately 3 percent of the general population and normally happens to people between 40 and 60 years of age and primarily to women. People with this condition have a very difficult time with sleeping for a long time due to the pain that gets worse at night and the restrictive movements or sleeping positions. It also happens to the person's non-dominant shoulder. There are three clinic phases one goes through when diagnosed with a frozen shoulder.

1. *The painful or freezing phase*: This takes place within the first four months or so. A patient will experience constant diffuse pain, especially when lying on it at night. The stiffness and limitations actually build up and gets worse as time goes on. If the patient tries to push it, they will feel muscle spasms. The patient might get so discouraged and depressed that they will start not to use the arm.

A good suggestion would be that if you have not seen any improvements with your physiotherapist or allied health worker, taking a break might actually be better than trying to push through the pain. Trying to fight through the freezing phase won't work. As I said before, this is a systemic issue, and one needs to let it run its course, while trying to maintain the strength and range of motion as much as possible.

2. *The frozen or stiffening phase*: It takes approximately between 4 and 12 months. The good news is that the pain starts to decrease or ease but the stiffness and lack of range of motion remain and can get worse. All movements of the shoulder can be affected, but it is the worse with external rotation. Keep in mind that if you are not using the joint due to the stiffness, the muscles don't get used, and may weaken or atrophy.

3. *The thawing or recovery phase*: This phase can last between 12 and 18 months. You start to gradually get back your shoulder range of motion, the pain is less and you will feel it mostly with movement, and you return to normal or almost normal.

Medical treatments are also possible in some cases. Sometimes surgery might be discussed, as a last resort, if nothing else helps. That can be done through manipulation of the joint by the surgeon under anesthesia, although it is less commonly done these days due to a risk of a fracture in the area. Another way is through an arthroscopic surgical capsular release, where the tight part of the capsule is loosened up by using a special probe. This is normally outpatient surgery, followed by physical therapy to decrease the risks of contracture and get the area moving. Results have been shown to be fairly positive.

Short of surgery, doctors can help you by a hydrodilatation injection, carefully injecting water and a local anesthetic into the joint to stretch out the capsule. This procedure is done via X-ray, so that the doctor can see exactly where to inject in the area. The studies show that the patient, who is awake for the procedure, can feel an immediate improvement in their arm. Following the surgery, the patient will need physiotherapy to continue to move the joint to maximize any benefits that were produced. Please discuss this option with your doctor and understand all the risks involved before attempting this type of surgery.

The symptoms of a frozen shoulder can persist until three years later, but for most people life returns back to normal in terms of function and movement after two years, and sometimes even without treatment.

You will start to compensate elsewhere for the lack of movement that you have in the shoulder, and you will not be a happy camper. So, get that problem seen by a doctor, ASAP!

Do I Have Calcium in My Shoulder?

Calcific tendinitis is a form of tendinitis, which is defined by having crystals, called *hydroxyapatite* (which is a crystallized calcium phosphate material) found primarily in the rotator cuff muscles of your shoulder, causing inflammation and severe pain. The condition has been known to be connected to and cause frozen shoulder, spoken above. It is normally a 1–2 centimeter calcium deposit found in the tendons of the rotator cuff. The most common place that it occurs is in the supraspinatus tendon. These crystals are normally found in patients who are between 30 and 40 years old, and diabetic. It is also commonly seen in women, and for some reason it happens primarily in the right shoulder. The good news is that it moves in a predictable fashion, and usually will go away eventually without any need for surgery.

There are three main stages here as well:

1. *The precalcification stage*: A patient doesn't normally feel anything in this stage as the calcium crystals start accumulating and depositing into the tendon and the connective tissue.
2. *The calcific stage*: There are two parts of this stage, the resting stage and the resorptive stage. Once the calcium has been deposited and calcification has been created, the resting period begins, which can last for weeks, months, or years. Officially this is not the painful period. Once you start with the resorptive phase, however, the pain begins and is the most painful part of calcific tendinitis.
3. *The postcalcific stage*: At this stage, the calcium deposits start to disappear and are replaced by the normal rotator cuff tendon. Due to this replacement, this is when people also feel a lot of pain.

How Do I Know I Have a Tendonitis to My Rotator Cuff?

Signs and symptoms of a rotator cuff injury may include:

- Pain or tenderness in your shoulder, commonly in the top, front or on the side, as well as your upper arm (sometimes all the way down to your elbow) when you make overhead movements.

- Shoulder starts clicking and/or an arc of shoulder pain when you place your arm at about shoulder height
- Pain when reaching behind your back, swimming or throwing movements
- Pain/weakness in the front part of your shoulder when you are combing your hair in the morning, tucking in your shirt, or putting your arm behind the passenger seat when you are backing up the car
- Pain posteriorly at night when sleeping on your affected shoulder
- Pain in the front of the shoulder when carrying something heavy, or bending your arm backward to put on a jacket
- Not wanting to move your shoulder, or cradling your affected side with your good arm (as in a sling)
- Loss of range of motion

As your shoulder tendonitis gets worse and worse, you might even have shoulder pain at rest.

Common Causes of a Rotator Cuff Injury

- *Lifting*: Lifting something heavy or quickly when your shoulder is not strong enough to lift that weight, or lifting something using an improper technique can place an unnecessarily huge strain on your shoulder. These actions might also excessively internally rotate or turn your shoulder inward, causing a pinching or stabbing sensation in the anterior or front part of your shoulder. This can cause enough pain to actually involuntarily let go of the weight that you were holding—especially with overhead movements.
- *Poor posture*: This is a very common problem! The majority of individuals don't seem to realize that they can acquire a rotator cuff injury from bad sitting or standing biomechanics. When you are in a forward sitting position and you start to hunch your back and slouch your shoulders forward, as you work in front of your computer or if you read this book in a slouched position in your chair (you wouldn't be doing that now, right?), you put a tremendous and unnecessary amount of stress on your neck and shoulder. This happens a lot when a person sits at the edge of their chair. Did you know that a forward head posture can contribute to a difficulty in swallowing as well as sleep apnea (sleeping with an open mouth)? We will get into how to better position yourself in chapter 5, which exclusively deals with posture.

- *Falling*: Falling is a traumatic injury. Placing an outstretched arm to stop yourself from falling can give you anything from a tear in your rotator cuff tendon or muscle, to a possible dislocation of your shoulder joint, to a fracture of a bone. Always have a medical specialist check you out before resuming any other activity or sport.
- *Repetitive faulty movements*: As previously mentioned, continuous movements, done incorrectly, can create serious pain and limitations to your shoulder. These are the injuries that can creep up on you, with your not knowing where and when they started and developed into full-blown injuries.
- *Age*: Although commonly occurring to people between the ages of 20 to 40 years old, a rotator cuff injury can be more serious and take longer to heal later in life. Normally, after 40 years of age, the normal wear and tear of everyday use can cause the collagen fibers that make up the tendons to break down and slightly pull apart. This makes them more prone to injury and degeneration. The average age for this injury is estimated approximately at 55 years old. In people over 70, 21 percent had shoulder problems that came from the rotator cuff.

It has been shown that shoulder pain is the third most common form of musculoskeletal injury behind low back and neck pain. But it doesn't have to be this way! If you strengthen your shoulder properly, using the correct exercises, then you will be on your way to healthy and strong shoulders.

- *Muscle imbalances*: There are 2 major ways of getting injured: It can be traumatic or a biomechanical injury.

A traumatic injury is pretty self-explanatory. Examples of traumatic injury include falling down on an outstretched arm and separating or dislocating your shoulder, or having a high-speed accident and sustaining a fracture of the scapula, clavicle, or humerus.

Biomechanical injuries, on the other hand, are the ones that come suddenly without an onset of injury. Some biomechanical injuries can come from sports related activities due to the extreme ranges of motion and excessive repetitive force placed on the shoulder. Such sports may include overhead pitching in baseball, performing the crawl or other swimming strokes, serving in tennis, repeatedly spiking the ball in volleyball, and so forth.

Other times the complaint might come supposedly with no warning at all to the person working every day in a sitting position in front of a computer at a desk. Some of my patients tell me the following: "I don't really know how it all began. One day I woke up and all of a sudden I felt this awful pain in my shoulder."

What most people don't realize is that an injury of this sort can come from everyday compensation of certain muscles or poor sitting habits, and not necessarily from just a traumatic injury.

By bringing your head and shoulders forward, as you would in an improper sitting position, you create a muscle imbalance between your big internal rotator muscles (pec and lat muscles) and your smaller external rotator (infraspinatus and teres minor) muscles. This would also create lots of tension in your mid-back region or rhomboid muscles area, due to all the straining they do to pull you back from a leaning forward position to a straight one. That would create some very tired muscles.

When the front of your body caves in, your upper back and shoulders are being overstretched. This creates a huge muscle imbalance, and with time, your internal rotators will become adaptively shortened, as well as your upper back and external rotators of your shoulder becoming quite lengthened.

Proper exercise routines can help put the "balance" back in your shoulder and help decrease some of the discomfort that you are feeling.

RRRRIP! TEARS IN THE ROTATOR CUFF

A torn rotator cuff is one of the most common causes of shoulder pain and disability. According to the American Academy of Orthopaedic Surgeons (AAOS), an estimated two million people in the United States seek medical help for a tear in their rotator cuff.

As you now know, when we speak about the rotator cuff, we are really speaking about the tendons that form a protective ring around the top part of the humerus bone—not about muscles at all. But these tendons do get torn, primarily in two ways.

A partial tear, also called a *partial thickness tear*, does not completely sever the attachments to the bone. These tears usually occur along the side of the rotator cuff, in the bursa or in the tendon. There are mainly three spots on the rotator cuff that you can have a partial thickness tear: 1) articular side tears, 2) bursal type tears, and 3) intratendinous tears.[1]

Articular side partial tears are the most commonly seen and involve tendon fibers found adjacent to the head of the humerus. Bursal-sided tears are less common, found in approximately 2.9 percent of the population, and they happen to occur at the area of the cuff that faces the subacromial bursa, the more superiorly located fibers. Intratendinous tears, which are found inside the fibers of the rotator cuff tear, make up approximately one-third of partial thickness tears and may occur alone or in combination with the articular and bursal type of tears.

There are three grades of tears: Small tears (less than 3 mm deep) and medium tears (3–6 mm deep) involve less than 50 percent of the tendon thickness. However large cuff tears are more than 6 mm deep and affect more than 50 percent of the tendon thickness.

For anything with under 50 percent of the tendon torn, surgeons will do what is called *surgical debridement*, which is the cleaning or removing of the necrotic or dead tissue from a wound by using a scalpel or scissors. This is the quickest and most effective form of debridement. With anything above the 50 percent range, surgeons will mostly opt for an outright surgical repair, mostly in the articular-sided region.

A complete tear, or sometimes referred to as a *full thickness tear*, is a tear or detachment of the rotator cuff tendon from where it originally attaches from. It has been shown that this kind of tear does not heal very well.

There Are Two Types of Rotator Cuff Tears

An acute tear occurs when someone experiences a sudden type of movement, like falling on an outstretched arm or lifting something real heavy with a quick jerking motion.

A chronic tear is the one most physiotherapists and other allied health professionals see more often. It is completely torn through, like poking a hole though a paper with a pencil. A tear of this kind happens slowly over time, and gets bigger and bigger after years of repetitive overuse movements.

Tears can happen anywhere on the rotator cuff, but the most common tendon to tear is the supraspinatus tendon. There are two reasons that this happens. First, a part of the supraspinatus lies between the humerus bone and the clavicle, therefore making it very vulnerable to being impinged and damaged. The second reason may be due to its blood supply. It has been shown a specific area, called the *critical zone*, of the supraspinatus tendon has a very poor blood supply.[2]

WHAT IS AN IMPINGEMENT SHOULDER SYNDROME?

Having an impingement syndrome in the shoulder is as common as someone saying, "I have sciatica," or "I must have shin splints." But what does having a shoulder impingement syndrome really mean?

Shoulder impingement syndrome has also been called *painful arc syndrome, subacromial syndrome,* and *thrower's* or *swimmer's shoulder.* It is really a condition in which the tendons of the rotator cuff muscles that pass through the subacromial space of the shoulder, which is located underneath the acromion process of the scapula and above the humerus, become inflamed or irritated.

There Are Really Two Types of Shoulder Impingement Syndrome: Primary and Secondary

Primary shoulder impingement occur when something goes into the already crowded subacromial space and pinches the rotator cuff and bursa. There is not a lot of room to begin with so with something extra in there, there is a higher chance that rubbing can occur, causing an irritation. An example of this might be a bony spur coming off of the undersurface of the anterior third part of the acromion, as well as the coracoacromial ligament—a condition that made Dr. Charles Neer, an orthopedic surgeon in the early 1970s, term the phrase *impingement syndrome.*[3]

A secondary impingement syndrome is the one that most people are familiar with. That is when a joint instability exists in the glenohumeral or scapulothoracic joint. The symptoms here are overuse syndrome of the rotator cuff and surrounding muscles from an increase of work that some of the muscles try to do (at the expense of weaker muscles) to try to stabilize the shoulder. An imbalance of these structures can cause a mechanical impingement of the rotator cuff. In certain patients with scapular instability, impingement has happened with an improper position of the scapula on the humerus, causing a decrease of scapular retraction and impingement of the rotator cuff.

Although both types of impingement injuries might look the same—you get pain when you raise your arm up—it is a very good idea to be checked out by your doctor or allied health professional, because the causes of each syndrome is completely different. For example, if your shoulder impingement is really due to a bony spur going into the subacromial space, verified by your doctor probably with an X-ray and an

MRI, then a surgical intervention might be the best and only way to help you. If there is no bony spur or other structure in the space and the weakness of the rotator cuff and surrounding muscles just decrease the space, then a proper exercise program to stabilize the joint and area might do the trick.

The subacromial space, which acts like a small tunnel, actually will change dimensions through movement of the arm. If you lift your arm to the side, the space in that area will actually decrease. Why does that happen?

The reason is the following: You have an area on the humerus where some bone called the *greater tubercle* of the humerus sticks out. When you lift your arm to the side, the greater tubercle naturally will go into the subacromial space, therefore actually decreasing the already narrow space to begin with.

Tendons pass through the subacromial space as well as a bursa, called the *subacromial bursa*. A bursa, a flat, fluid-filled sac located over a bone, has the purpose of letting the tendons slide properly and reducing any friction on the tendons. If the tendons do not biomechanically slide properly on that bursa, the space is decreased, and the tendons will irritate the bursa causing a bursitis.

Keep in mind that all the other muscles also attached to the scapula need to work together and in balance to have proper biomechanical movement of the arm and shoulder. However, when the tendons do not work properly and are out of sync or balance, problems begin. Abnormal scapular movement and function is called *scapular dyskinesis*. An imbalance of the muscle pulling on the scapula can irritate the bursa and cause it to inflate.

Some examples of muscle imbalance that can cause poor biomechanical movement include lack of strength in the infraspinatus, teres minor and posterior deltoid that can create weak external or lateral rotation of the humerus. A weak serratus anterior muscle can cause a decrease in upward rotating and posterior tilting of the scapula. This can cause anterior tipping and some winging of the scapula, which is really bad. That, in turn, due to the lack of space available, will pinch the tendons, causing them to become irritated and inflamed. A tight posterior capsule can flatten out the posterior aspect of the capsule itself, causing the humeral head to come forward and upward in the glenoid fossa. This abnormal position can pinch the tendons even further, causing pain and discomfort. This is called an *impingement syndrome*.

What I would like to point out at this point in time is that we do not really care which specific structure or group of subacromial structures are affected or impinged. Trying to exactly diagnose it is not so easy. What is more important is determining what biomechanically abnormal movement caused it and giving the proper exercises to help it.[4]

Is My Injury Due to Stress at Work?

I believe that stress, due to a hectic work life, personal issues, or any other unpleasant situation can create a psychological response that can suppress your body's immune system. Therefore, stress affects the entire body. If an area is already weak or strained, like your shoulder or your neck, stress can lead to more tensions and spasms. I find in my practice that people will rarely complain about stress in their strong areas—for example, I don't feel any tension in my forearms, elbows, or thighs when I am stressed or anxious. We almost always complain about the stress that we feel in our necks and shoulders. I believe that if we strengthen and stabilize these areas, the feeling of stress will lessen. It is important to manage stress before the tension and anxiety puts you in a downward spiral.

Just remember that there is no one way that one can handle one's stress, because everyone is different. I know that some people get rid of their stress by doing yoga; others curl up on the couch to read a good book or they take a nice long hot bath. My best way is to release stress and anxiety through exercise. You can always do some kind of exercise—from walking, to dancing with your loved one, to playing soccer—that can help and release anxiety. It really doesn't matter what you do as long as it is something that you love.

Some people don't even know how to relieve their anxiety in the simplest ways known: just by breathing properly. When we become anxious, we tend to breathe in shallow breaths or even hold our breath. Sometimes we are not even aware of it. When you take shallow breaths, you actually bring in less oxygen than normal, making you even more tense and anxious, and pain in your shoulder and neck can only get worse. Just practicing a bit of deep breathing can help you a lot. Here is how you can do it properly:

Make sure you are sitting up properly in your chair. Posture is important as you will see in chapter 5. Place your hand on your stomach just above your waist to monitor your breathing. First you should start by exhaling through your mouth. Then breathe in slowly through your nose, pushing your hands out with your stomach. This will guide you in breathing slowly and deeply, creating a sense of calm and relaxation. Exhaling takes a little longer to do than inhaling. Keep practicing slowly until you get the hang of it; then you will not need to use your hand anymore. Once you feel that you have mastered this technique, try doing it in a lying down position. Deep breathing exercises can relax you and really help you to go to sleep at night.

How Should I Sleep When I Have This Tendinitis Bothering Me?

It has been said that there is no ideal way to fall asleep. Each person has their own way. The easy answer is to not sleep in the position that is not hurting you. Of course, that is easier said than done. Sleeping in a bad position might actually make your injury feel worse. So here are some helpful tips:

Start by sleeping on your opposite side—the one that does not hurt. If your right shoulder hurts, sleep on your left side and vice versa. Place a pillow in between your arm and body to prop up your arm and not allow it to fall forward, keeping it in a neutral position as if you were in a sitting position. This will allow your shoulder muscles to relax. Also, try to get a pillow thick enough to keep your head aligned with your spine, so that your head is not bending either way.

Try not to move so much when you are sleeping. One trick I tell my patients to use is to place a long or body pillow between their legs (added bonus: this might relieve some of the stress in the low back). The pillow length might discourage you from thrashing back and forth in bed, hurting yourself in the process.

Another tip might be to not sleep on your stomach (as I do) when you have shoulder pain. The stomach position does not allow the shoulders to stay in a stable position and can create muscle spasms that wake you up (cursing silently) at night. If you prefer to sleep on your back, sleep with a small pillow on the back of your shoulder to bring it a little forward. This will help your rotator cuff muscles relax. Make sure your neck is also supported, because if it is not, your position can place a compression on your nerves, creating a feeling of numbness or tingling that shoots down your arm.

In terms of a mattress, try to pick one that isn't too hard or firm, or that isn't too soft. A good mattress that will conform to your body without creating too many pressure points works best. If you are in the store shopping for one, lie down on them and try them out. You will know right away which one feels the best for you.

Is My Rib Cage Related to My Shoulder Pain?

Yes it most certainly is. The rib cage, which is connected to your thoracic spine, doesn't have as much mobility as your neck or lower back, but it is very strong and stable. The rib cage and the scapula make the scapulothoracic joint. Therefore, because of this union, proper and efficient movement of the scapulothoracic joint really depends on the position of the rib cage that the scapula slides along. If your rib cage is not in its ideal place, that will in turn change the position of the scapula, making it slide a little out of whack and creating an impingement problem. Patients with shoulder impingement problems have less thoracic spine mobility in extension (bending backward rather than forward) compared to normal healthy people. Increasing the thoracic spine extension and general mobility of your thoracic spine will help increase your breathing, as well as decrease your shoulder and neck problems. The thoracic spine is normally stiff when the back muscles are weak and overstretched due to bad posture.

GETTING HELP

Should I see a physiotherapist, osteopath, or a chiropractor for my injury?

This is probably the number one question that patients ask their friends, colleagues at work, and most definitely their doctor. Although it is a simple question, it does not have a clear-cut answer. Although I am a physiotherapist, I will try my best not to be biased with my answer. The first step is to explain what each practice does for the patient.

Osteopathy is really a holistic form of manual, hands-on therapy, which treats acute, chronic, and systemic problems that are happening with the body. An osteopath deals with musculoskeletal injuries as well as visceral or organ problems. What my colleagues at my clinic have explained to me is that an osteopath doesn't treat a specific area like a shoulder or back, but treats the body as an entire unit that is suffering an ailment and tries to get the balance back to the body (the way it was before the injury occurred). They see the body as an amazing machine that can and should be able to fix itself from even a traumatic event. However, when the body is overwhelmed from trying to cope with the injury, it may need a helping hand. That is when the osteopath will come in to help it along.

I have seen our osteopaths here at the clinic do some amazing things for patients who could not be helped otherwise. Osteopaths can do mobilizations, but can also perform manipulations if necessary. Some of the techniques are so gentle and specific that sometimes you can barely feel that anything has been done, but you start to feel better, sometimes almost immediately (depending on the condition).

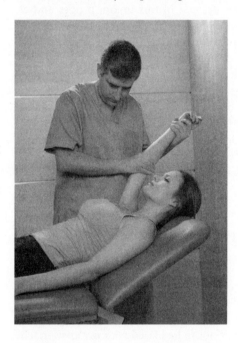

An osteopath moving a woman's shoulder.
Holbox/Shutterstock

Everyone has heard of a chiropractor. Actor Jon Cryer plays a chiropractor on the hit TV show, *Two and a Half Men*. But what does a chiropractor really do?

Chiropractors believe all of the patient's issues can be traced directly back to the misalignment of the spine. This misalignment causes a deterioration of health. It is their belief that if they can properly correct the alignment of the spine through spinal adjustments, the rest of the body will follow, and the patient's problems will get better. They are well-known for their manipulations, especially in the neck or lower back.

Okay, if these professions use their hands to fix issues, what does a physiotherapist do?

Physical therapy or physiotherapy is a health-care profession whose job is to correct impairment and disabilities of the patient and try to give them back the quality of life that they had before they had their injury. There are many branches of physical therapy, but the one that deals primarily with muscles and tendons is the branch called *orthopedics*.

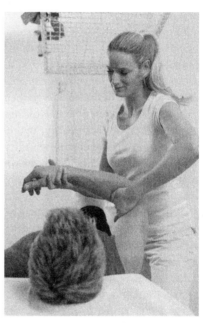

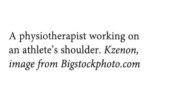

A physiotherapist working on an athlete's shoulder. *Kzenon, image from Bigstockphoto.com*

What you see when you go to a private physiotherapy setting is really an ortho-out clinic. (*Ortho-out* is short for orthopedic outpatient, meaning the patient comes in, gets their treatment, then they go out; they can leave the facility.) An ortho-in facility would be a hospital, with a patient not being able to leave the facility—for example, a hip or knee replacement requires an ortho-in facility.

Physiotherapists are health-care professionals who diagnose and treat people of all ages—from little ones to seniors and all walks of life. The youngest person I ever treated was eight years old; the oldest one was ninety-six. My category of physiotherapy is in the orthopedics, or musculoskeletal area, where the physiotherapist helps a person with an injury that would limit the patient's ability to do their everyday functional activities. I work closely with the medical doctor who has referred clients to me. The PT or physiotherapist's job is to listen to a patient's history and physical examination to establish a management plan to get them better and back to their sport or everyday life as fast as possible. We might differ from others in that we are strong believers of specific exercises to help with range of motion as well as strength, flexibility, and balance of the region in question. To us, proper functional movement is central to making the patient healthy again.

Our manual therapy skills comprise mobilizations and, if needed, manipulations, strength and range of motion exercises, pain-reducing modalities (ice, heat, electricity, ultrasound, and host of others), as well as educating the patient about what they have, how they got it, and a management plan for how to get better.

It might sound like I am avoiding the question as to which therapy— physical therapy, osteopathy, or chiropractic—is better, so here is my two cents: I do not believe that one profession is "better" than another. I rather subscribe to a belief about which therapist is better than another. A more experienced individual might be better than another therapist straight out of school. All therapists who you might see have the same goal in mind: to get you better. There are many different methods, but everyone's goal is still the same: to get to that point. I would say then, pick a practitioner who has a good reputation, who you like, and most importantly, who you trust. You can never go wrong that way.

Let me also explain what the difference is between a mobilization technique of a joint and a manipulation.

By using hands-on manual therapy, a joint mobilization is really a type of passive movement of any joint on the skeleton. It can be done by a chiropractor, osteopath, or physiotherapist. During the mobilization technique, if the patient is not happy and wants it to stop, the patient can actually stop the movement from happening voluntarily by contracting his or her muscles and the practitioner will also stop the movement.

Patients who have a sensitive nervous system really do well with mobilization techniques, because these techniques are light enough to not over-stimulate the nervous system and produce unnecessary muscle spasms.

A manipulation, on the other hand, is a completely different method. It is a thrust technique, done at the end range of the joint's range of motion. Here is the main difference: The patient really has no control over a manipulation. The patient cannot stop the manipulation midway through the movement. With a joint manipulation, you might hear a popping or cracking sound. If you ever wondered what that really is, it is called *cavitations* of the synovial fluid of the joint. It is a little complicated to explain, but basically by pulling the joint capsule apart you momentarily deform the joint capsule, creating a decrease in pressure of the joint capsule. That's why you get that temporary relief. When a manipulation is done properly, it can give immediate relief to the patient suffering from musculoskeletal pain.

There are obvious contraindications with manipulations done improperly. They are infrequent, but they can range from disc herniation or rib and vertebral fractures, to strokes and vertebrobasilar accidents (VBA). My advice is to always speak with your practitioner first before a manipulation, so that you are comfortable with the technique.

When Should I See the Doctor?

You should see your doctor as soon as possible if you are feeling any kind of shoulder pain or discomfort or if you are having difficulty moving your arm in any direction. A doctore is always the first professional you should seek. The first doctor you see is probably your general practitioner or your primary care physician. As the name implies, a general practitioner is a doctor who doesn't have a specific specialty, but has a general medical practice in which he or she deals with all illnesses. Normally, after carefully listening to your story, the doctor might refer you to a different kind of doctor, a specialist.

There are different kinds of specialists, such as a physiatrist (rehabilitation doctor) or an orthopedic surgeon. But it is usually best to start with your general practitioner.

A physiatrist in the medical world is a doctor of physical medicine and rehabilitation. This doctor works in a section of the medical field that specializes in "physical" medicine, such as medications and physiotherapy. They have a special type of training in diagnosing and treating of the bones, muscles, and nerves of the musculoskeletal system. Their goal is to do what they can to get you better—without surgery.

Physiatrists' specialized training gives them the edge in understanding the biomechanics of the shoulder and surrounding regions, and how to properly take care of the rehabilitation of a shoulder problem or any type of musculoskeletal injury in the body. These doctors' goal in their treatment is to get you as pain free and functional as soon as possible. This is exactly the goal of a physiotherapist, so what a great team you would have if you had both of these people in your corner.

A physiatrist can either be a medical doctor or MD, or a doctor in osteopathic medicine or a DO. Some physiatrists even get further training, learning how to give injections such as epidurals and facet blocks of the spine.

An orthopedic surgeon is a doctor who is trained to use surgical or nonsurgical methods for treating trauma to the musculoskeletal system, sports injuries, degenerations, infections, or anything else that can't be treated conservatively. They are the ones who take care of muscle, tendon, or ligament tears; shoulder joint dislocations; and everything that might be related to the musculoskeletal world.

A patient will normally go through surgery when everything else has not worked. For example, if you have a shoulder issue, and after physiotherapy treatment or any other type of rehabilitation suggested by your doctors has not worked, then surgery is the way to go. In my opinion, a surgical intervention should be the last thing that should be tried. You must realize that after surgery, you will still take a while to recover fully, still need physiotherapy or other treatments to give you the full range of motion, strength, and flexibility needed to go back to your daily routine.

Call your doctor or your allied health professional (e.g., physiotherapist, athletic therapist, osteopath) if your pain is lingering and does not seem to be going away. Don't let the problem drag on, saying that it will leave any time soon. Pain is your body's way of telling you that something is wrong, so listen to your body. Ignoring it or just telling yourself that you just have to accept it, without first getting it checked out, might cause more harm than good.

If for any reason you can't see your regular doctor, and your condition is still very painful, you can go to the emergency room at your local hospital. The doctor there might prescribe you some anti-inflammatory medication to help get rid of your pain.

If you have seen the doctor and can't determine what exactly the cause of your shoulder pain is, he/she might send you for some diagnostic tests. These might include the following:

MRI (magnetic resonant imaging) scans: The MRI is a diagnostic examination technique that uses medical imaging to see the structure and function of the body. It uses a combination of radio and magnetic waves to create two- or three-dimensional pictures of your body. The good thing about an MRI is that it does not involve exposure to X-rays or any other form of radiation.

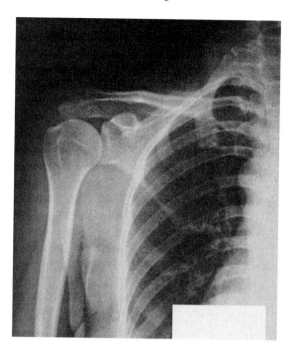

An X-ray of a shoulder.
itsmejust/Shutterstock

MRIs are primarily used in understanding neurological conditions, problems of the musculoskeletal system, which include muscles and joints, as well as tumors and heart abnormalities. Two issues that you should be aware of about the MRI machine is that it can get a little claustrophobic when you are in it, and there might be some noises as the test goes on (but nothing to worry about). You also have to lie still when the test is proceeding. The test normally lasts for 30 to 60 minutes.

The MRI machine is safe because it has no known dangers and produces no side effects. Since it does not use any radiation, you can repeat the test without any danger.

X-ray: An X-ray machine is a diagnostic tool that uses high-energy electromagnetic ray beams that pass through the specific area of the body, and take images or a picture of the structure in question. When the energy beam does not go through a structure, it will appear on the X-ray film as being black. If a structure, such as a bone, absorbs the energy, it appears white on the X-ray. Different structures in the body absorb the rays differently, and they will therefore show up like different and distinct structures on the X-ray film. For instance, in a normal X-ray picture, most soft-tissue structures, like muscles or ligaments, don't appear on the film. It would be more beneficial to use an MRI machine or even a CT scan (described below) for those structures.

Although too many X-rays can be harmful for you, it is still a safer option than a surgical intervention. An X-ray machine is an invaluable device in the world of medicine, and a great invention.

CT scan: A CT scan or a CAT scan is really known as a computer axial tomography, which uses special X-ray techniques to take multiple detailed images or "slices" of the body. A computer then joins all those multiple pictures together to form a cross-sectional view of the area that the doctor wants to see. It has much better detail and clarity than a conventional X-ray machine. A CT scan can take these "slices" of internal organs, blood vessels, bones, as well as soft tissue, like muscles and tendons.

It is an effective device for looking at problems of the spine, hands, feet, and all the skeletal structures because it can show fairly clearly even the tiniest bones, as well as the muscles and small vessels around it. CT or CAT imaging can be imagined as if you slice thin pieces of bread from a whole loaf. When all the pieces are placed together, with the help of a computer, the result is a very multidimensional view of the structure that needs to be seen.

Okay, So What's the Real Differences Between an MRI and an X-Ray?

While an MRI and X-ray machine both take images, there are some fundamental differences between them.

Function: An X-ray is primarily used to determine if your bone is broken or fractured or dislocated. It can also detect slipped discs in the spine, as well detecting diseased tissues. An X-ray can only see bone or other dense tissue, and that's it.

An MRI, on the other hand, is used for soft tissue injuries—for example, ligament or tendon injury, spinal cord injury, brain tumors, and so forth.

Cost: An X-ray will normally cost approximately $70, whereas an MRI can start from $1,000 and run all the way to $4,000 (if a contrast dye is being used).

Time: An X-ray usually takes a couple of seconds, whereas an MRI scan can normally run for approximately 30 minutes.

Radiation exposure: An X-ray creates exposure to radiation, whereas an MRI gives off no radiation.

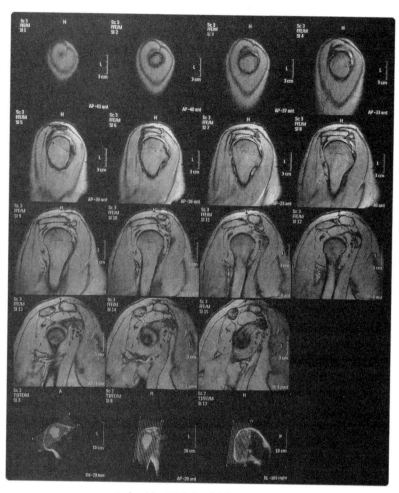

A shoulder MRI. *Sarah2/Shutterstock*

Details in visualizing soft tissues: An MRI can definitely see soft tissue, and even in better detail than a regular CT scan. An X-ray cannot see soft tissue, which appears as a shadow on the image.

Image plane: An MRI machine has the ability to produce an image in the plane it is put in. The machine has the ability to change its plane of viewing without actually moving the patient. With an X-ray machine, you have to move the patient.

Versatility: An MRI is much more versatile than an X-ray and is used for a wide variety of medical conditions, whereas an X-ray is really limited to just the few body conditions that it can see.

The difference between an MRI and a CT scan is that an MRI can take pictures from every angle, whereas a CT scan can only take pictures horizontally. If you are looking for the difference between normal and abnormal tissue in the body, MRIs are generally more detailed and clearer. The cost of a CT scan is about half the price of the MRI, and takes about 5 minutes for a CT scan to be completed versus the 30-minute MRI scan.

A major advantage a CT has over the MRI is that it is able to see bone, soft tissue, and blood vessels together, while an MRI can only see the soft tissue clearly. CT scans can also see the different tissues much more clearly than the MRI, especially if a contrast dye is used. It can also create a higher image resolution.

A person who has a metal implant in their body can still get a CT scan, but patients with metal implants, pacemakers, or tattoos are not allowed to get an MRI because the resulting image might become distorted or the patient might become injured.

An MRI machine can create a claustrophobic situation, and medication to alleviate anxiety and induce relaxation are sometimes prescribed beforehand because the patient must be totally still during the test. That isn't necessary with the CT scan.

Ultrasound: Ultrasound or diagnostic ultrasound is another diagnostic medical imaging technique use to see contractile tissue (e.g., muscles, tendons) and any pathological issues. During a diagnostic or medical ultrasound, a medical probe that sends sound waves is passed over the injured area. Due to the fact that sound waves pass poorly through air, some ultrasound gel is applied. The sound waves that are emitted go to the injured part of the body and reflect back to the ultrasound transducer and sent to the machine's scanner, which are then taken, processed, and changed into an image. The images that come back to the ultrasound machine are viewed, analyzed, and stored for later review. The unique aspect with ultrasound is that it can work with real-time images, therefore showing movement, function, as well as the anatomy present. This in turn further helps in diagnosing the problem. Ultrasound images are useful in diagnosing tendon and ligament sprains and strains as well as tears in the muscle.

Again, no X-ray or iodizing radiation is involved in the ultrasound procedure, which is painless. The other advantage with ultrasound is that it is portable and much less expensive than an MRI or a CT scan, usually ranging from about $100 to $1,000, depending on the country.

Arthrogram: An arthrogram is a diagnostic test using an X-ray and a contrast type of material (usually a dye, water, or plain air) to take an image of a joint. This is another option that doctors have when an X-ray is not complete enough for a proper diagnosis. The procedure is normally done using local anesthesia. This procedure is primarily done for tears of any kind, including rotator cuff tears. If you have a normal rotator cuff, the dye or water will stay within the tissues, but if you have some sort of tear, the liquid will start to leak out of the tissues. Arthrograms can either be done as a diagnostic tool or a therapeutic one. A cortisone injection for your shoulder that a doctor might suggest to you is considered a therapeutic arthrogram.

Although there are many other tests that your medical doctor might ask for, these are some of the major tests that you might be asked to go through. Ask your doctor what would be the purpose of you going through the specific test suggested.

CHAPTER TWO SUMMARY

A primary shoulder impingement is an inflammation or irritation of the tendons of the rotator cuff muscles. Secondary impingement, the more common form, results from instability in the joints of the shoulder caused by the imbalance.

A tendinitis results from minor, "incorrect" movements done repetitively over time; it is most common between the ages of 20 and 40.

Bursitis results from an bursa irritation caused by an imbalance between two opposite sets of muscles; the irritation keeps the tendons from sliding easily and results in pain and weakness.

Tendinitis is marked by pain or tenderness in the shoulder and/or along the upper arm, especially when reaching overhead or behind, carrying a heavy weight, or even doing nothing at all. Calcific tendinitis results from the formation of crystals in the rotator cuff muscles.

Frozen shoulder, or adhesive capsulitis, is pain and loss of motion in the glenohumeral joint, the main shoulder joint.

Rotator cuff tears may be partial thickness, which do not sever the attachments to the bone, or full thickness, in which the rotator cuff detaches. Rotator cuff tears may result from sudden movement in which both the motion and force of the motion are excessive and acute.

Health-care practitioners who treat shoulder problems include osteopaths, who perform joint mobilization; physical therapists who prescribe targeted exercise movements for strength and range of motion, pain reduction, and prevention; and surgeons, who become involved when other modalities fail.

3

The Pain

"Everything hurts."

—Michelangelo

Mary doesn't remember falling. To this day, she cannot tell you whether she tripped over a flaw in the sidewalk, or blacked out for some reason, or was nudged by a passerby and lost her balance. All she knows is that she was suddenly splayed out on her side on the pavement, with her shoulder underneath her, in such pain that she knew she couldn't move. The friend with whom she was on her way to the movies phoned 911 on the cell phone, and an ambulance took the significantly injured Mary to the nearest emergency room.

Paul remembers his traumatic injury only too well. A passionate hockey player, he plays in an amateur neighborhood league for the over-40 crowd. In one Saturday afternoon game, Paul was set to bodycheck his opponent with the puck, missed, and slammed into the boards instead—shoulder first. He couldn't believe the pain.

You fall, slam, crash, bang, get hit—and your shoulder takes the brunt of it. These are traumatic shoulder injuries; both the damage and the cause are obvious.

Far less obvious are the nontraumatic injuries to the shoulder. One day, the shoulder feels a little stiff, so you massage it a bit and go back to what you were doing, assuming that the discomfort will pass. A couple of days later, the discomfort is back. It's worse. You stretch your arm this way and that. Better—sort of. Back to what you were doing. Ouch! It still hurts. Your movements are constrained, limited. But what can you do? You've no idea how this happened. You didn't fall, didn't plow into something, didn't collide with anything. Yet the pain, when it happens, is hot and sharp. Each time it strikes, it startles you with its intensity.

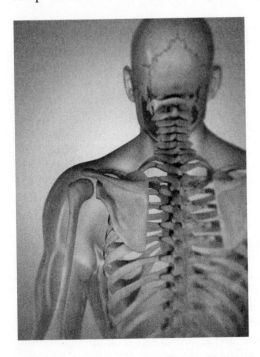

Shoulder pain. *Sebastien Kaulitzki/Shutterstock*

It is the kind of pain that builds over time—just as the injury to your shoulder undoubtedly happened over time. How did it happen? Most likely through posture—the position of your body or the way you carry yourself when standing or sitting. If you have a desk job or work at a computer all day, if your job consists of lifting hefty objects or of reaching overhead a lot, if you spend a lot of time behind the wheel of a car or have a pack on your back or a tote bag slung over your shoulder all day, over time, any and all of these situations can end up affecting the rotator cuff and causing you those sudden, dramatic bursts of shoulder pain.

The bad news is that since you can't recall a reason for the pain, you think it will go away by itself. It won't—as you well know by now; it's why you're reading this book. So how can you deal with the agony and get yourself on the road to fixing your shoulder quickly, confidently, and effectively?

PAIN IS A SIGNAL

The very first thing to do is to acknowledge the pain and accept it for what it is—a signal that something is wrong with your shoulder. The Marys and Pauls of this world have no trouble recognizing the signal; they know something is horribly wrong.

Pain is one of the body's best ways to communicate between the brain and the injured area. It is the body's way of protecting itself from causing real harm to itself. Pain acts as a warning signal that tissues are being damaged, and will make you remove yourself from the source. What would happen to our fingers if we couldn't feel pain when placing our hands over a hot stove, or accidently touching a sharp object? We would definitely have suffered unnecessary damage to ourselves. The purpose of pain is really to protect you, not hurt you. Think of it as your body's internal alarm system.

On the other hand, pain creates severe discomfort and unpleasant sensory and emotional feelings. Every person experiences pain differently, from being able to handle the feeling to being totally incapacitated from it.

The two major categories of pain can be classified as acute and chronic.

According to Segen's medical dictionary, acute pain is "a normal, physiological and usually time-limited response to adverse (noxious) chemical, thermal or mechanical stimulus."[1] Acute pain normally happens immediately and lasts for the first 24–48 hours. It is usually created by a particular injury or physical ailment that can be treated once we figure out where the problem is coming from.

Acute physical pain can come from a sprain in your shoulder, caused by quick movement, or a muscular strain caused by lifting something way too heavy that your muscles were not ready for. Making a wrong move can cause acute pain to shoot through a certain area of your body, like your shoulder. You can experience acute pain caused by everything from stubbing your foot in a door, to having a major accident.

Subacute pain is a little harder to define. It is between an acute pain and a chronic pain, yet it is more common than people realize. We often see people in subacute pain in the clinic.

Subacute pain normally begins 48–72 hours after the initial injury and can last for months if not taken proper care of. In this stage, after the inflammation part has happened in the acute initial phase, the body starts to do the repair work on the injured area. It will normally start working on the "construction site" by laying down some new tissue in the form of collagen. In the beginning this collagen is very "immature" and is a little disorganized. It takes, on average, 6–8 weeks to fully mature the region. We decide that an area is doing okay or has healed when it has reached a level that it can handle the load it did before the injury. It has its full range of motion and experiences no pain.

Chronic pain begins at approximately six months or so. Studies have shown that someone who is suffering with chronic pain has experienced changes in their personality, with sharper than normal mood swings, from increased depression as well as feelings of anxiety, to suicidal tendencies. Stress and pain can become a vicious cycle that is hard to escape. When you are in pain, you feel more stressed and anxious. The anxiety and stress can cause your muscles to tense up, which will increase the pain even more. Therefore it is always better to see a health specialist sooner rather than later; the concept "it will go away on its own" is not something to rely on.

Pain affects men and women differently. Women generally are able to experience more pain, be much more open in conversations about the effects of pain, and are better able to cope with pain than men.

Here are a few different examples of shoulder pain that we frequently hear about:

"I feel something in my shoulder, but I can live with it. It must mean that I am getting old, and I just have to get used to it."

"My shoulder is not that bad, I just feel the pain when I sometimes wake up from sleeping on it."

"Every time I reach for something, my shoulder gets so painful that I can't move my arm at all afterward."

These are examples of different degrees of pain, from mild to potentially severe. It is important to realize that even if your shoulder is not preventing you from performing your daily activities or sport, a problem still lingers that you need to take care of, before it becomes worse. Do not ignore your pain.

One other thing to know is that there are mainly two types of shoulder injuries: traumatic and nontraumatic or biomechanical injuries.

Traumatic injuries are the ones where trauma has recently occurred, as in a person that fell down and landed on their shoulder. It is painful right away and the individual knows how the injury occurred. It produces an acute type of pain.

A nontraumatic or biomechanical injury is more difficult to diagnose. This is the type of injury that starts gradually, with no apparent traumatic event occurring. "I don't know when it started. I started to feel my shoulder ache slightly, but I ignored it. I thought it was going to go away. As time passed by, however, the pain moved from my shoulder all the way up my neck and between my shoulder blades, and I didn't know what was going on."

The injury might happen due to bad sitting at your computer or other postural positions. As time passes by, this problem can eventually become more painful in nature. But for those of you self-diagnosing shoulder pain as "just an ache"—and maybe deciding that what you really need to do is pop a bunch of pills, wait it out, or, as some people believe, give the shoulder a bit of a workout—hold it right there. Putting off dealing with the pain you feel now leads to one certain result—much worse pain down the road, and very possibly much more damage to your shoulder. Be clear: This pang of discomfort is your body's telling you that something is wrong—and resolve to get expert help in dealing with it.

CAN TAKING MEDICATIONS FOR MY SHOULDER PAIN HELP?

Yes, medications prescribed from your doctor can definitely help you in your combat to relieve your shoulder pain. But taking medications is only a part of the game plan to fix your shoulder and keep it healthy and happy. Also, medications can produce some side effects, so you will need to speak to your doctor before trying anything. It is significantly better to have a team around you than to try things yourself. It is also important to find a doctor who has some expertise in shoulder problems. Your family doctor might refer you to an orthopedic shoulder specialist as well as a physical therapist, osteopath, chiropractor, or any allied health professional who can help.

I would also suggest not being afraid to get a second opinion about your condition if you are not sure, or if the medication is not working. This is very important if you are considering surgery.

Once the doctor has given you a diagnosis, some of the medications or treatments may include the following: muscle relaxants, which will decrease the spasms that you might be feeling and relax the muscle, and anti-inflammatory medication, which can help the body get rid of the inflammation that is presently there.

CORTISONE SHOTS

You have heard about cortisone shots. What do they do exactly?

Cortisone shots are injections given specifically for joints, like your shoulder. They have a corticosteroid medication and a local anesthetic. Cortisone shots are normally performed in the doctor's office. They are supposed to help relieve pain and inflammation in your shoulder due to tendonitis or bursitis around the rotator cuff area. You would normally receive a shot if the treatment that you are receiving, through physical therapy, modalities such as ice or heat, medications, or electrical modalities, is not really helping the situation.

To help understand if the limited range of motion is coming from the shoulder pain or from weakness, a cortisone shot is normally injected in the subacromial space that we spoke about earlier. If the anesthetic gets rid of the pain and allows you to move your shoulder properly, then the problem probably is some form of rotator cuff disease. If your shoulder, however, still feels weak after the injection, then a rotator cuff tear is probably the problem.

After you receive your cortisone shot and the anesthetic wears off, 4–6 hours later, you may feel some discomfort for the first few days. The corticosteroid in the cortisone shot should begin to kick in and relieve the pain and inflammation after one to two days. In my practice, I have seen that cortisone shots can provide relief from inflammation and pain for up to several weeks or even more. On other patients it might be much less—like a week. And for some people, a cortisone shot might not help at all.[2]

The number of cortisone shots is limited due to the potential side effects of the medications. As well, having multiple cortisone injections in the same area can weaken your shoulder tendons. Your doctor may wait up to two months before another cortisone shot is performed. The maximum number of shots given is from three to four shots. This is a lifetime limit. If the first cortisone shot does not seem to work, a second one may be given to ensure that it was given in the right spot. There are some side effects with cortisone shots, so always clear them with your doctor. Side effects can include the following:

- Increased pain may occur during the first few days after the injection.
- The tendon in question can start to degenerate.
- Your skin color might change.

- Infection at the site (rare) may develop.
- If you have diabetes, you may get an elevated blood sugar level.

Because of the injection, your rotator cuff tendons may be a bit weaker than normal, so no strengthening exercises should be done for a couple of days. You also should not do any contact sports after a cortisone shot, because an already damaged rotator cuff may get more damage.

There are many different types of modalities that your allied health practitioner can use—from ultrasound, shockwave therapy and iontophoresis, to interferential current, and everything in between.

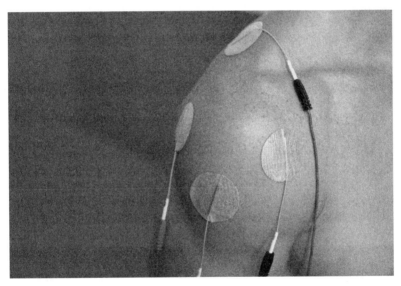

Physical therapy using an interferential current. *Kattitude, image from Bigstockphoto.com*

COLD SHOULDER

Until you can get an appointment to see the doctor or physical therapist, what can you do about the pain? There's a simple answer to this question, and it's amazing how many people in pain refuse to accept the answer. It's ice. What you want to do is numb the pain. Yet for some reason, this seems counterintuitive to a great number of people.

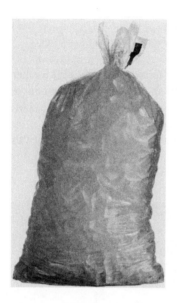

Bag of ice.
Steve Heap/Shutterstock

Take the case of a patient I'll call Mike. He doesn't like ice. Actually, Mike doesn't like anything cold (except beer). When he phoned me about what he dubbed "searing" shoulder pain, and I told him to put ice on the shoulder right away, Mike had reservations. The shoulder was in spasm—very painful—and Mike just sensed that heat was what he wanted. So he stepped into a hot shower, turned the water up as hot as he could stand it, and then held the detachable shower head directly on the shoulder. Ahhhh. Mike felt the spasm abate. His whole body relaxed. He felt fantastic. He turned off the water, stepped out of the shower, and was just starting to close the shower door when he felt that same searing pain shooting through his shoulder and down his arm. It was almost unbearable.

But it changed Mike's mind. Maybe, he thought, I can freeze the whole area till I don't feel anything anymore.

What a concept, Mike!

Why Is Ice Better than Heat in These Painful Situations?

Ice is an anti-inflammatory agent, just like Advil or an aspirin. It reduces most inflammatory activity from occurring at the injury site. In contrast, heat, unfortunately, is an inflammatory agent.

You want as much inflammation in the area of pain to decrease as quickly as possible—not to increase. Ice has been shown to be better than heat for any initial injury to the musculoskeletal system, especially in the first 24–72 hours.

What really is inflammation? It is really an automatic body response to an injury in the body. It is like the body's garbage truck that removes the extra or waste products that are still around after an injury has occurred. Although inflammation is the first stage of the healing process, and is very necessary for your injury to eventually improve, the body tends to go overboard with inflammation production. This leads to problems if all that excess inflammation is allowed to continue to take place and swelling is allowed to stay and accumulate in the injured region. This swelling will prevent normal oxygenated blood from reaching the injured tissues. If that is allowed to occur, this will lead to a condition called *secondary hypoxic injury*, in which the cells get further injured or even perish due to a lack of oxygen supply. When cell death occurs, the inflammatory process begins again. This is why ice (with compression, elevation, and rest) is great for decreasing the inflammation, swelling, and hypoxia (lack of oxygen) stages.

Ice can also reduce and even inhibit muscle spasms from occurring due to the elevated level of pain.

When applied to your specific region, ice lowers the temperature of that area, therefore decreasing the amount of inflammation that the body produces in that region.

Can I Ever Use Heat?

I do not recommend placing heat on an area that is painful, tender, or even very sore. With that said, there are some times that some heat can be beneficial to you. Sometimes a good time to use heat may be when you wake up in the morning and you just want to loosen up a part of your body. (That is why taking a nice hot shower in the mornings is so refreshing!)

By the way, the most efficient way to warm up a body part is . . . drum roll, please . . . exercise! Yes, that's right, exercise increases your body core temperature the quickest (and the safest).

So if you are looking for just a quick loosening up of the body, then heat is your answer. If you are feeling some kind of distress or discomfort, then again go with the ice. You won't go wrong.

Best Ways to Use Ice on an Injury

1. Crushed ice placed in a Ziploc bag with a wet towel around it
2. A bag of frozen peas or vegetables with a wet towel around it
3. Commercial cold packs
4. Ice cold creams
5. Ice massage

These are definitely not the only methods of putting on ice. There are many different other ways, from cold whirlpool treatments or ice bucket treatments, all the way to different types of cold sprays.

In fact, Mike is exactly right about what ice can do—get you to the point where you feel nothing. Here's how to do it:

Fill a sandwich-sized plastic bag—like a Ziploc—with ice cubes. Wrap the bag in a wet towel—yes, wet—and apply it to the point of pain. You can do this by lying down and setting the apparatus on top of the shoulder, or by lying down with it under your shoulder. Or you can strap it to you with an elastic bandage, easily obtainable at the local drugstore and probably sitting in your medicine cabinet or first aid kit right now.

Why a wet towel? Because it is a far better conductor of the cold than a dry towel and thus works far faster and more efficiently.

The pain-reducing process goes through four stages: cold, burning-cold, aching, and numb. Numbness means you have frozen the pain, and you feel nothing. That is what you're shooting for. Once you get there, remove the icing apparatus.

How long will it take to achieve numbness? That of course will vary from person to person depending on the depth of the pain, your own pain threshold, and how well you put together the icing apparatus and apply it. But as a general rule, it will probably average between ten and 15 minutes for most people to reach that frozen state of nonfeeling.

If possible, ice the pain every couple of hours. Of course, this is a tall order for most working people, but try to do it at least twice a day—morning and night.

Then, be absolutely sure that you do not do any kind of physical activity that could affect the shoulder. Certainly do not go back to whatever you were doing when you first felt the pain—whether it was playing tennis or reaching up to retrieve a book from an upper shelf. You may indulge in activities that don't affect the shoulder; go for a run if you like, but no push-ups, no weight lifting, no catch with the kids.

And whatever you do, see a licensed medical practitioner—even if the pain goes away. (It will likely come back.) It is important to have a diagnosis of your of your injury, nontraumatic or traumatic, so you can move on from there.

Unless surgery is required, the moving on will focus on physical therapy.

When Not to Use Ice

Do not use ice on your skin if you are suffering from the following:

Cold allergies: Ice allergies are extremely rare, affecting 1 to 2 percent of the population. You might experience hives, some joint pain, or nausea. The removal of the ice bag will help clear this up.

Reynaud's phenomenon: This is a condition that makes it much more difficult for the blood to reach certain parts of your body, because it makes the blood vessels under your skin tighten, called *vasospasm*. If that happens, no blood makes it to the designated area, which will turn blue and feel very cold. This is not a good sign. This is seen in the fingers and toes area. If you have not tried ice before, keep checking the area frequently for this occurrence.

Severe large open wound: Infections become a primary problem in this area, and you don't want to put anything on it that is not sterilized. Make sure you cover or have someone cover up the large open wound with a sterile dressing.

Decreased sensations to ice: Any one with a lack of sensation in a specific area should not be placing heat or ice in that affected region.

Circulatory problems (i.e., hypertension): Cold should not be placed over circulatory-compromised regions of the body. Patients with circulatory problems can make their problems even worse with ice, causing a vasoconstriction effect over already nutritionally deprived regions, which in turn would exacerbate the situation.

Diabetes: Patients with diabetes have poor or decreased circulation to their extremities in varying degrees. When ice is placed over these compromised areas, local blood flow decreases. That is the last thing you want to do in an area that is already not getting enough blood flow.

When to Use Ice

Acute injury: Ice should always be used in the first 48 hours. If heat is placed on the injury site, an increase in inflammation will occur, worsening the condition.

Analgesia/painful area: Ice is always recommended when pain is involved. It will reduce the velocity of nerve conduction, as well as slow the metabolism, reducing the cell's need for oxygenated blood and reducing additional cell death. If an area is numb, you won't feel the pain.

Reduce muscle guarding/spasm: Studies have shown that ice is better for muscle spasms than heat. Ice creates a higher threshold for a nerve action potential or stimulus to occur, making a muscle contract. Heat has a lower threshold, creating spasms much more quickly.

There are definitely more excellent pain-reducing modalities that can be used for your injury. Please consult your doctor or health professional for any questions that you might have.

MOVING ON—AND KEEPING THE PAIN AT BAY

Your physical therapist will clue you in on the operating principle of working on any muscle—namely, that you must achieve range of motion before strength, and you must achieve power before endurance. (At least, that's what the therapist should tell you. If he or she suggests strengthening exercises first, change therapists.) The theory behind this is simple and obvious: You don't want to strengthen the impairment of limited range of motion; you run the risk of locking in the limit. So the first aim of the shoulder-fixing process is to achieve full range of motion. The process starts out easy, may proceed slowly, and often requires patience.

Patience is precisely what Ashley lacked. The quintessential type-A personality, she worked for a Wall Street firm and held to the view that time was money. So when her therapist, a colleague of mine, started her on range of motion exercises and warned her not to tackle the strength exercises till later, Ashley balked. The ranges of motion exercises were so easy; it seemed a waste of her precious time to bother with them at all. Instead, she went headlong into the strength exercises of the program.

The first exercise she tried called for lifting a weight in front of her as she raised the shoulder upward. Hmmm. That was hard. What if, Ashley thought, I just swing the weight upward with my body? Swing! That worked. Again: Swinging! Ashley felt a jolt of electricity through her shoulder, and she crumpled to the floor. She could not move her arm at all. When she was able to get up and make a phone call, she asked her doctor to prescribe some heavy medication for her. He did so, told her she was lucky because she might have torn her rotator cuff completely, and advised her to "listen to your therapist."

Of course, like Ashley, everyone wants to get back in the game quickly. But the truth is that there is no precise way to predict with any certainty how long it will take an individual to regain his or her full range of motion. Each case is different. Your therapist will ask to see some simple movements as a way of trying to gauge the degree of flexion or extension you may be missing. That is, your therapist will evaluate the degree of bending and straightening you are able to do. He or she may ask you to raise your arm as high as you can and then judge, for example, that you're "missing" 30 degrees of flexion and will assign exercises that help you regain full flexion. How long it takes to do that will depend on your age, your diligence in doing the exercises, your pain threshold, and more.

The "Overdoing It" Delusion

Too much diligence can be as bad as too little. Olivia held to the belief that more is better. When her therapist assigned her to do range-of-motion exercises once a day, she instantly assumed that doing them three times a day would get her better three times faster. Morning, afternoon, and night for a week, she kept at it, until by day eight, she was in so much pain from the overworked spasms that she could barely move her arm at all. Olivia had to wait till the spasms relaxed and the pain disappeared before starting again—from scratch. This time, she did it gently, patiently, and exactly as her therapist prescribed.

Not until range of motion has been solidly achieved should you attempt any kind of strengthening exercise. Physical therapists typically define "solidly achieved" as 70 percent to 80 percent of full range of motion, the absolute minimum for initiating strengthening exercises. Ideally, I recommend waiting till 100 percent of full ROM has been achieved, but at the very least, I would say you don't want to start the strengthening process till you have 80 percent of full ROM. It isn't just that you run the risk of more pain; you also run the risk of real damage.

A steady patron at the gym where I work—I'll call him Howard—is a case in point. Tall, with a powerful physique, Howard looks more like a bodybuilder than like a production executive in an entertainment company—which is what he is—an appearance stoked by the weight lifting to which he is partial. "No shoulder exercises at all till the pain is virtually gone," I advised him. "If you must work out"—and Howard shows up at the gym just about every day—"stick to cardio exercises and work your leg muscles. But don't do anything that affects or uses the shoulder. Certainly no weight lifting. It would really endanger your recovery."

Howard stayed away from the gym for a week. Then I noticed him on the jogging track and later, taking a spin class on the stationary bike. Fine. I wasn't at work a few days later when Howard passed by the weight room at the gym and decided, in his words, that he would do "just a couple of sets of bench presses." It would be "no big deal," he thought. "Nobody will even know. It should be okay."

It was on the third rep of his second set that he heard the rip in his shoulder. Howard screamed. A guy on the next bench sat up and grabbed the weight out of Howard's hand as Howard cradled the arm against his chest. The doctor later confirmed that Howard had suffered a complete muscle tear of his supraspinatus and scheduled him for surgery the following week.

Surgery is the last thing you want. The bottom line? Listen to your pain, and do what your therapist tells you—no less and no more.

HOW EATING RIGHT AND DIFFERENT TYPES OF THERAPY CAN HELP

It is not a real secret that eating healthy food will get and keep your muscles stronger. It will also help injured muscles get stronger more quickly. You do not need a special diet to have your muscles stronger. Eating a balanced diet will give you all the energy you need to go through your day. Keep in mind that having some irritation or inflammation of a joint, muscle, or tendon can slow down the healing process of the area. Therefore, just like exercise or massage, some foods will aid specifically in the healing of tendons. I will try to be a little bit more specific about what you need to acquire some good tendon health.

As noted earlier, tendons are extensions from muscles and attach on a bone. They are made from dense connective tissue, which feels like a cord, when you touch it through your skin. Due to the fact that tendons have a limited blood supply, and are always working and under constant tension, it is difficult for them to repair quickly when a strain or tear has occurred.

Foods that have high active enzymes can really give that jolt that tendons need and help them with the healing process. Examples of these superfoods are pineapple and papaya. These two foods have some specific enzymes (called *bromelain* and *papain*) that are very active types of enzymes in the bloodstream and can really contribute to helping the body get the injured tendon healed more quickly.

Another important food contributor that aids in healing is vitamin C. The reason why vitamin C is so great is that it helps with the production of collagen, which is most abundant in the tissue of a tendon.[3] Great foods that contain vitamin C include broccoli (now you know why mom was right!), berries, oranges and other citrus fruits, tomatoes, peppers, Brussels sprouts, and spinach.

Vitamin E is another great antioxidant that can help reduce inflammation. It is a fat-soluble vitamin and having too much of it can become toxic, so please don't overdo it. I would rather you get vitamin E in food rather than in a supplement. Vitamin E works together with vitamin C to create the formation of collagen. Vitamin E is interesting because it can only be absorbed if there is adequate fat in your diet. You can find vitamin E in such foods as nuts, seeds, avocados, and green, leafy vegetables.

Vitamin B6, manganese, and zinc are other vitamins and minerals that can also contribute in the improved health of a tendon.

Tendons have quite a bit of calcium in them; therefore, having some foods that are rich in calcium can have a positive effect on the healing of the tendons. Milk products, which we all know have plenty of calcium, as well as fermented milk products like yogurt or buttermilk, can also help.

Some nondairy foods also have a lot of calcium in them. These include my absolute favorite, salmon, as well as sardines, spinach, peas, broccoli, Brussels sprouts, and bok choy. Basically, any food that is high in collagen or any other component of connective tissue is good for tendon healing. Therefore meat is another good source, but fish and poultry are even better sources because they have much more connective tissue in them. It has been also shown that any soup that has any joint or any bone tissue, for example, pho, which is Asian tendon soup, is also a good choice.

Believe it or not, some juices can actually make your condition heal more slowly. Fruit juices have a very high amount of sugar, and high blood sugar can actually increase inflammation. I suggest that you refrain from drinking them, as they will not help with the nourishment of the body after a strain or sprain of a tendon. What I would recommend, however, is vegetable juice, especially cold juicing. This actually preserves the active enzymes found in the vegetables, and still gives the great concentrated nutrients. I also highly suggest that you use the guideline of drinking approximately eight cups of water during the day.

Some supplements have also been shown to help with the healing process. Arnica, a popular herbal remedy, has been proven to help treat tendon and joint pain. In the form of oil, it is normally applied and rubbed into the injured area. Arnica has shown to decrease swelling and inflammation and can reduce the amount of time it takes for the tendon to recover.

Rue is another herbal remedy that can be used to relieve pain related to your tendonitis, or other muscle injuries. An anti-inflammatory component in rue has been shown to strengthen the capillaries in the body.

There has been a lot of talk about omega-3 in the news—and for good reason. Found in fish, omega-3 fatty acids have been found to increase the body's anti-inflammatory response to tendonitis, as well as having many more health benefits. I really like it, and try to incorporate it in all my food, whether as an oil or in my salmon.

Lastly, cayenne pepper, although mostly known as a food seasoner, can also cause blood vessels to expand. This can help the body bring more blood flow and more much-needed nutrients to the injured tendon area, helping promote healing.

There are a lot more nutrients out there, like turmeric and quercetin, that have anti-inflammatory properties and can help with the healing.

Make sure you check with your doctor before you start any regimen for healing.

CAN ACUPUNCTURE REALLY HELP WITH MY SHOULDER?

Acupuncture comes from very old traditional Chinese medicine, dating back more than 3000 years ago, which involves correcting over almost 2000 points in the body that are connected with pathways of energy, normally called *meridians*. The energy points are called *qi* or *chi*. These points on the body have bigger concentrations of nerve sensations and blood vessels than other parts of the body. The whole point of acupuncture is to fix or balance out any blocks in the qi meridians by stimulating these points and therefore clearing the way for the energy to go through the body, and thereby helping the body get itself better.

We all know that there are needles involved in acupuncture. These are really super thin, disposable needles made of stainless steel that are inserted through the skin and are then twisted in a particular pattern on the meridians. The particular pattern that the needles are placed in will depend of the injury and what the patient's symptoms are. The needles are then left in for approximately 30–40 minutes. Different people get different sensations from acupuncture. Some might say that they feel a pricking sensation with some warmth or an aching feeling. While some people might experience a sense of calm and relaxation, to the point of falling asleep, others might experience an increase of energy in their bodies.

Acupuncture helps shoulder and any other type of pain by stimulating the release of opioids, which are painkilling chemicals, as well as by stimulating adenosine, which is a natural painkiller and anti-inflammatory components.[4]

What is the difference between acupuncture and cortisone shots? It really comes down to location. When a cortisone shot is used, it is placed at the injured site, which will cause some discomfort to the patient. Acupuncture needling is placed above and below the injury, therefore not aggravating the irritated area at all. Unlike cortisone shots, acupuncture needles do not deliver medicine. Acupuncture is very effective for helping shoulder tendinitis and other painful injuries. In case you were also wondering, acupuncture is safe with very few side effects.

WHAT ABOUT YOGA?

Yoga is something that started thousands of years ago in India. It combines exercise, stretching, controlled breathing, and meditation, all in one. When done consistently and faithfully, this form of exercise can really reduce pain and discomfort by stretching those areas that are super tight, and inflexible. It also does wonders to decrease the stress and tension in the body that a person feels every day.

Sometimes doing a yoga pose places additional stress on the joint, especially the most famous pose of all, the downward dog. It really comes down to incorrect technique—for example, placing all the weight on the wrists instead of also placing some of the weight equally on the hands. If you find that your fingers are lifting off the floor, the technique would probably give you some discomfort. Try placing your weight on your entire hand and grip the mat with your fingers. This will develop the strength in your hands and fingers and, at the same time, will take the stress off your joints, thereby decreasing the risk of developing a tendonitis.

Some specific yoga poses can actually strengthen the shoulder region. For example, instead of doing a full downward dog, try doing a half downward-facing dog, which is a modified pose done on the wall. Try placing your palms flat on the wall, approximately at shoulder height, and walk so that your feet are under your hips. Now try to bend forward with your head between your arms, with your spine being approximately parallel to the floor. As you keep both hands on the wall, try turning your arms inward and keep a slight bend on the elbows. Lastly, turn your upper arms outward, so that the head of your humerus bones are being worked in the shoulder region.

Some other poses that you can try, like the warrior 2 pose or virab-hadrasana II, which will really strengthen your stabilizing rotator cuff muscles. Another yoga shoulder exercise that is beneficial with shoulder tendinitis is called *marichyasana*, which is a seated twisting pose.

One last note on the downward dog: If not done correctly, it can actually add stress to the shoulder and create a tendinitis, if you are not doing it properly. Try and keep your external rotators engaged, by keeping your elbows straight but not locking them.

SHOULD I DO PILATES?

Pilates is a form of exercise developed in the early 1900s by Joseph Pilates, who was a physical culturist from Germany. He believed that the physical and the mental were connected to each other. We know now how true that is. After studying different forms of exercise and fitness, he developed a method of exercise himself, "Contrology" (stemming from the word *control* and the Greek word meaning logic). Pilates began with mat work and developed a series of exercises done with springs and other different resistances, which he eventually turned into functional equipment that he used when he helped disabled soldiers in World War I. After the war, he started to teach his style to professional dancers, world-class gymnasts, actors, musicians, and high-society New Yorkers. In the 1980s his teaching went from athletes to Hollywood celebrities, and eventually to the general public.

Pilates is a system that can increase flexibility, and muscle strength as well as endurance—not only in the abdominals, as it is popularly known, but also in the entire body. The most famous apparatus, the reformer is really a rolling platform that is secured by springs. It is quite unique in that

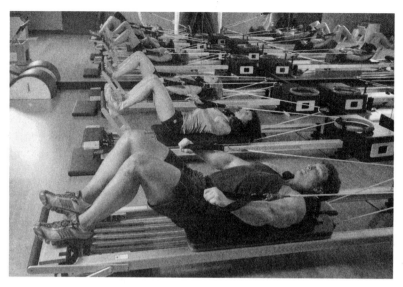

Demonstration using Pilates reformers. *Gino Santa Maria, image from Bigstockphoto.com*

in many exercises you lie down flat against the machine. It does not place any compression on the spine, because it is in a gravity-free plane. Pilates works on proper spine and pelvis alignment, proper breathing technique, and most definitely works on your core muscles. It is really amazing for someone who does not want to bulk up and get massive, but rather look lean and defined with a killer posture to boot, You won't see an elite dancer or a Cirque du Soleil performer in a hunched-over position.

The Original Six Principles of Pilates Training

1. *Centering*: According to the Pilates method, the way to control your arms and limbs is to develop your core, which is the center of your body. Referred to as your "powerhouse" area, all movements should start from this area and move outward. This makes all other movement so much more efficient and much less energy draining. The secret to developing this powerhouse region is to try to do all the exercises while maintaining a neutral pelvis. A neutral pelvis position is exactly the same thing in every human being: It is the alignment of your ASIS (Anterior Superior Iliac Spine or your hip points) and

the pubic bone in line with each other in the coronal plane (which divides you in half, making the front and back of your body).

2. *Concentration*: In order for the Pilates training to be successful you must have intense concentration and focus in what you are doing. This is why I am a big believer in one-on-one training. Normally in a Pilates studio, it is quiet. No blaring music, no human distractions. It is really you and the instructor. Of course, there are two-on-one classes, and even group classes, but those are not the same as one-on-one sessions. The instructor cannot be everywhere, looking and spotting if anyone is cheating the exercise (and there will be times that you yourself do not know that you are cheating). The most efficient way to getting your money's worth is to have an instructor who basically stands above you and kindly correct your movements—for example, reminding you to bring your head back, relax the muscles on your face and neck when you do your abdominal exercise, and so forth. Trust me; you will feel a big difference. You are so focused on what your teacher is trying to get you to do, that there is no way that you have time to look at something or someone else.

3. *Control*: With concentration comes control. Pilates is always quoted as saying "the reason that you need to concentrate so strongly is that you can be in complete control of all your movements. Your movements must be smooth and fluid."[5]

4. *Flow*: Pilates always aimed for an elegant flow of proper movement through specific precision. Once that high level of precision has been attained, then smooth flows of movements should occur from one exercise movement to another. This builds stamina as well as strength. Therefore Pilates builds smooth, controlled flowing exercises from your strong core.

5. *Precision*: Pilates teachers really emphasize that their students focus on doing one perfect movement rather than performing a lot of half-focused ones. The point is that these exercise movements that are super-hard in the beginning eventually become second nature and natural. This will also carry into grace and economy of movement in everyday life.

6. *Breathing*: This last Pilates principle is the one that newcomers say is the hardest to master—proper breathing. Pilates himself referred to breathing as a form of "bodily house-cleaning with blood circulation."[6] He believed that full inhalation and exhalation was the key to the body getting cleansed and making you feel invigorated.

Pilates always stated that full-forced exhalation was the key to complete exhalation.[7] Pilates breathing requires the client to breathe deeply into their back and into the sides of their rib cage. When they then breathe outward or exhale, they are told to contract their deep abdominals and pelvic floor muscles, and keep this position as they inhale. Another important point is to combine your breathing with the exercise movements that you are performing. Above all, Pilates want his clients to learn how to breathe properly.[8]

CHAPTER THREE SUMMARY

- Pain is a signal; pay attention to it.
- Apply ice for pain and let it work through four phases from cold, to burning-cold through aching, to numbness—the goal.
- Full shoulder activity rest is advised until pain is gone.
- The exercise therapy progression is to achieve range of motion before strength; achieve power before endurance.
- Ideally, you should regain ROM fully—100 percent—before initiating strengthening exercises; at the very least, regain 80 percent of ROM.
- Always put ice on an injury, never heat.
- Crushed ice in a Ziploc bag with a wet towel around it is the best way to apply ice to an injury.
- If you are not sure whether to use ice or heat in your situation, always choose ice!
- If it is your first time using ice, make sure you do not have any contraindications to using it.

4

The Fix

"Perseverance is failing 19 times and succeeding the 20th."

—Julie Andrews

The number one, best way to end your shoulder pain is to fix your shoulder impairment, and the number one, best, and fastest way to do that, barring surgery, is through a program of exercises.

That's what this book is all about. It offers you a program of exercises that fix what's wrong with your shoulder and thus end the pain. This is exercise as therapy—another Greek word, meaning cure or healing, something that I'm sure sounds particularly attractive to you right now. That program is coming up in the very next chapter, chapter 5.

But in chapter 7, I will also offer you different programs of exercises, routines you can practice for a lifetime to keep your shoulder strong and stable and thus able to avoid further impairment and later pain. These are exercises for prevention, and are just as important as, and even more useful than, exercises as therapy.

But whatever end result you seek, whether it's to fix what has gone wrong or to maintain a sound, strong, stable condition in your body, exercise exists in a context—its own frame of reference. It is essential to understand the parameters of that context before you undertake any exercise program, and that's what this chapter is about.

Specifically, the context consists of three things: the warm-up, the way we count or measure exercises—as sets of repeated movements separated by rest, and the stretching that ideally takes place after the exercises. Here are the why and wherefore of each.

THE WARM-UP

Advisable at any time for any kind of exercise, the warm-up, which is too often neglected, is particularly important in ensuring you don't simply re-injure the area that you've already hurt and fixed.

When you warm up a muscle, it means precisely that you are raising its temperature. Raising the temperature in turn means that you can contract that muscle and its surrounding area more forcefully. The warm-up also drives oxygenated blood into the shoulder; this raises your blood pressure just a bit and thus also speeds up your heart rate. When you dial up your heart rate in that way, you get the heart pumping the maximum amount of oxygen throughout the body while at the same time eliminating all the waste products created by the work your muscles have done up to this point; it means a "clean slate" for your workout. The warm-up will also prime your nervous system, getting it ready to respond to the demands you're about to place on it during the intensive portion of your workout, and so it can direct your body's actions more effectively.

But a proper warm-up doesn't just get you going. Warming up can also postpone your fatigue limit. When your body is really ready for an intense workout, it can last longer than if you had started cold.

And of course, a good body warm-up helps prevent pulling or over-stretching the muscle. Muscles that are warmed up before an intense activity are more pliable and looser. They can more easily absorb the force the exercises exert upon them.

So think of the warm-up as the pregame activity before the real thing. In my view, your warm-up routine should take about 20 minutes, on average, depending on your needs and your level of fitness. Once you've completed your warm-up and are primed and prepared, your muscles feeling toasty-warm and eager to get to work; your heart, lungs, and nervous system are on the mark and waiting for the starting gun. Then and only then are you ready for your workout.

REPS, SETS, AND REST

Gym talk. It goes something like this: "How many reps do you do? How many sets of how many reps? How long do you rest?" But it isn't as arcane as it sounds, so let's try to translate and explain it.

Simply put, reps—the universally accepted shortcut slang for *repetitions*—are the number of times you perform a movement. Ten reps of front dumbbell raises means you raise and lower the dumbbell ten times. The lift up plus the lowering down together count as a single repetition.

Actually, there's a little more to it than just up and down, for both movements in a single repetition are important. Doing both of them right is important, both for gaining all the benefit possible out of your exercise routine and for staying safe. And unfortunately, one phase of the rep tends to get all the attention while the second is typically neglected—in my view, with very serious, adverse results.

Specifically, there are two phases to a single weight-training repetition. The concentric phase is the "harder" part: It is the lifting or pulling motion in which the muscle gets shorter, and it should be done explosively—with proper form, in one to two seconds. That explosiveness is what recruits the maximum number of muscle and tendon fibers in order to increase strength.

Then comes the eccentric phase of the rep, the phase in which the muscle gets longer. All too often, we apply little if any effort to this phase. Instead, we let gravity take over and more or less allow the weight to drop in what is basically a wasted movement.

This is a mistake, in my view. I don't think the eccentric phase of the rep should be a wasted movement at all. In fact, it is my belief that a number of rotator cuff injuries could be mitigated or avoided entirely if the eccentric phase of a repetition were properly strengthened. Perform the eccentric phase in a slow and controlled manner over three to four seconds, and it will strengthen your muscles as they lengthen. It's the way many professional athletes and Olympic athletes train, both for sustained strength in every phase of every movement and to decrease the chances of injury.

The reason is simple: Paying equal attention to both phases of a repetition makes you balanced. In my view, *balance* is the single most important word in the entire physical therapy universe because it is the single most important thing a body can be. If you are balanced in strength from every direction, with proper flexibility and range of motion, you will not get injured. That is why doing the repetition correctly, attending to both its phases, is more important than the number of repetitions you might do.

A set is the number of repetitions of the exercise you perform without stopping. If you lift a weight ten times, then stop and take a break, you have completed a single set of ten repetitions. One way to determine the number of repetitions you should do is to push yourself to a point of momentary failure of the muscle—that is, to keep on doing reps, *maintaining proper technique*, until you simply cannot do one rep more. This is a good way to increase strength gains in your muscle.

Alternatively, most exercise programs, such as the ones I present in this book, set forth a goal for each exercise—a specific number of sets of a number of reps that are advisable for maintaining strength and fitness through performing the particular exercise. As you will see, ten repetitions is a fairly common goal for a set, and when you see that an exercise program calls for "3 × 10" of a particular exercise movement, that means you're being asked to do three sets of ten repetitions: ten reps of the movement followed by a break, then another ten reps, another break, and another ten reps.

Three sets of 10 reps is by no means the only program advised for an exercise routine, but it is the most commonly practiced, and it is the mainstream methodology for weight training. True, in Olympic lifting or power lifting, fewer sets and fewer reps with heavier weights are common, and some research suggests that one set of exercises might be just as effective as three sets, but "three by ten" continues to be the norm, and I'll be using it as a goal for exercises in this book as well.

Let me explain why. Why 10 repetitions instead of 4—or 14? And why three sets instead of six—or instead of the one set the research claims may be just as effective.

The answer is that different frequencies of repetition produce different results. Fewer repetitions—typically, anything less than seven—affect muscle strength. More repetitions—say 12 to 20—work on the muscle's capacity for endurance rather than on its strength. Therefore, eight to ten repetitions comes down somewhere in the middle between strength and endurance, theoretically providing a benefit to both—a low enough number of repetitions to boost your rotator cuffs endurance and develop shoulder stability, while also constituting few enough repetitions to increase the strength and power of your shoulder muscles.

What you don't want to do is a lower number of repetitions with higher weight, because that raises the possibility of too much stress on the rotator cuff—and therefore of doing more harm than good. We want to get your shoulder as strong as possible, but we want to be as safe as possible while we are doing it.

Similarly, three sets, with a rest break between sets, constitute a solid middle ground between a sufficient number of reps to be effective and keeping the muscles from getting exhausted and therefore strained.

Keep in mind that when working out you should not be in pain when you are doing an exercise. If you do feel pain, you need to make a change in your routine. Either decrease the weight, rest longer, or do fewer sets. Working out should be enjoyable, not painful. When it is enjoyable, you keep on doing it, and that's what will help you realize amazing gains in a safe and effective way. And by the way, yes, people will notice.

STRETCH!

Stretching is good for you and makes you feel good. It is one of life's pleasures and one of the best remedies for just about anything that ails you. Done right and done every day, stretching is one of the best things you can do for yourself, and it is certainly the perfect end to any exercise routine.

For one thing, stretching is just simply healthy for the body. Done regularly, stretching can help you maintain range of motion and flexibility throughout your lifetime, no matter your age. It counters the muscle-shortening effects of long hours of sitting in an office or of bad posture, and that means fewer and less acute aches and pains.

It is why I recommend stretching every day, even if just once a day. Of course, there are days when you simply cannot. But don't let the lapse last; try to start up again the next day. After all, it's not like stretching your body requires any special equipment or clothing; nor does it take up a whole lot of your day, although it isn't something you can zip through.

The American College of Sports Medicine (ACSM) recommends stretching each of the major muscle groups for at least 30 to 60 seconds every time you stretch, and I agree. As a number of studies confirm, quick stretches—of 15 seconds or so—simply do not give the muscle enough time for optimal lengthening. One study done in 1994 found that holding a stretch for 30 seconds was just about optimum—as effective as holding it for 60 seconds and considerably more effective than stretching for 15 seconds or not stretching at all.[1] Still, 30 seconds per muscle group doesn't add up to a whole lot of time, and done properly, stretching is an investment that will pay you back handsomely.

What constitutes proper stretching? The truth is that there are many ways to stretch—at least half a dozen different techniques—each with its own name and purpose—from dynamic to ballistic to active isolated and more. The easiest and least complicated type of stretch is the static stretch. As the name implies, it's all about putting a muscle in a stretch position and holding it—static—for a period of time.

Here's how: Assume the stretch position for the muscle, begin the stretch, and when you feel a gentle pulling, stop pushing. Hold the position for at least 30 seconds, then *slowly* release. Rest for 15 to 30 seconds, and then repeat.

The stretch can feel a bit uncomfortable, but it should not be at all painful. If you feel pain, stop immediately and decrease the pressure. Do not for a moment suppose that if you push harder, you will get better results. The opposite is the reality: You might end up hurting yourself instead of giving yourself relief.

And there should be no bouncing in static stretching. Bouncing happens in ballistic stretching, and in my view, bouncing or moving too quickly into and out of a movement can push a stretch to the point of causing injury.

I don't mind admitting that I normally listen to my music on my headset when I do my stretches. It helps pass the time—both the time for stretching and for the breaks of at least 30 seconds I give myself between stretches. Stretching makes me feel great, and I find that the feeling of well-being is best achieved when I do a stretch three times for 30 to 60 seconds, so that is what I typically recommend to my patients and it is what I suggest to you.

Warm-up, the count, the post-workout stretch: These are the elements of any exercise program, whatever its purpose. Our purpose is to fix your shoulder, so let's turn to that now.

Stretching after an exercise workout helps maintain range of motion and aids in preventing injury. Static stretching is recommended, using a 3×30–60 formula, with 30 seconds of rest between sets.

I believe that an exercise-based treatment is the number one, best, and fastest way to heal most impairments of the shoulder, barring surgery. In this chapter, we will go through some the most essential exercises that you will need to help with your rotator cuff. These strengthening and range of motion exercises will have a direct positive benefit to your rapid rehabilitation of your rotator cuff. I will show you how to perform each exercise in proper form. These are by no means the only exercises that you can do to strengthen your shoulder, but these are the ones that I share with my patients on a daily basis. Now, I want to share them with you. Enjoy!

RANGE OF MOTION (ROM) EXERCISES

The purpose of these ranges of motion or ROM exercises is to reduce stiffness in your shoulder as well as increase flexibility and give you your full range of motion, which is needed in order to perform your daily activities. If your shoulder joints feels stiff and painful, move them gently through their range of motion. Do not go too much into your level of pain, just enough that you feel some tension or stretch, without being in pain. Also move slowly into the exercise and do not bounce. Never force the movement. Make sure you breathe throughout the exercise; holding your breath won't help.

Perhaps the most important of all the points made here is to STOP exercising if you are experiencing extreme pain. It is possible that you might have gone too far into the movement.

Supine Stick Flexion

Lying on your back, take a broomstick, or any stick you have, with both of your hands. Keep your knees bent to protect your back and place your feet on the floor. Keep your arms shoulder width apart and your arms straight. Letting the noninjured arm do all the moving, bring the stick toward and above your head and toward the floor, as far as you can. Please do not force the movement. Bring the stick all the way back to your knees.

Your goal: 3 sets of 10 repetitions

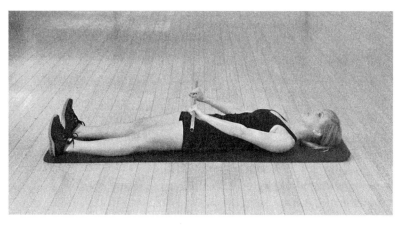

Beginning position of shoulder stick flexion

Ultimate goal: To be able to bring the stick all the way back, so that both of your arms are touching the floor completely. There is no major pain or discomfort in your injured shoulder.

Watch out for: Make sure the stick stays straight, and that one hand is in line with the other hand. Both arms should be moving in the same speed and at the same level. Also, don't hold the position at the end. It might cause a greater irritation than needed. Move into the position, hold for a maximum of 1 second, and then move back to the beginning of the exercise.

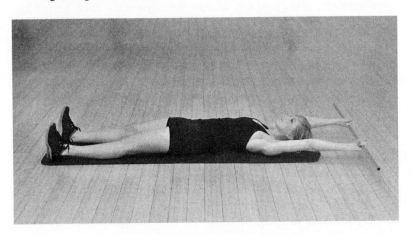

End position of shoulder stick flexion

Bent Over Arm Swings and Circles, or Pendulum Exercises

Bending forward from your hips, place your unaffected hand onto a chair or stable surface for support. Now let your injured arm hang. Gently, let your arm swing forward and back in a straight line. Don't force your arm, but try to be as loose as you can, allowing gravity to pull your arm forward to the ground.

Once you have done that for 10 reps, try the same movement, but now you will let your arm swing across your body or from left to right.

After you tried moving your arm from left to right, try the same thing, but in a circular motion moving in a clockwise direction.

Once you have completed 10 circles one way, try the same thing in the opposite way, this time rotating in a counterclockwise direction.

Your goal: 2 sets of 10 repetitions for each movement

Watch out for: Make sure you are always holding onto something to protect your back. If your back is acting up, try another exercise to get the range of motion you are looking for. This exercise should almost be relieving to your shoulder. If pain increases, recheck your position, or stop altogether. Finally, once you attain no resistance when performing the exercise and you have gotten your full range of motion, you can stop doing this exercise altogether because you attained the goal of the exercise: Performing it with no pain in its full range.

Standing Front Wall Walking

Standing in front of the wall, at arm's length, let your fingers do the walking. Using your fingers start, "climbing" up the wall comfortably until you cannot climb more. Relax your arm and start again.

Your goal: 3 sets of 10 repetitions

Watch out for: Make sure that you are standing close to the wall, slightly closer than an arm's length apart. Remember: this is a ROM (range of motion) exercise, and not a strengthening exercise; don't hold the position at the top. Also try not to arch your back or twist your body to get more range. Try maintaining proper position and mechanics throughout the movement. There is literature out there that suggests holding this position for 30 seconds, but this might in-

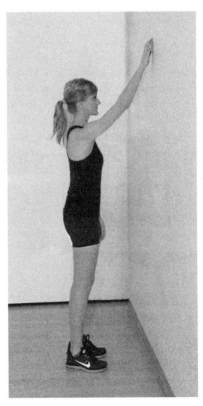

Standing front wall walking

crease irritation in the shoulder. I would prefer performing the movement more frequently than holding it.

Standing Side Wall Walking

This is the same exercise as the Standing Front Wall Walking exercise,
  but now you are standing to your side, perpendicular to the wall, at
  arm's length away again. Again, using your fingers, start "climbing"
  the wall as high as you can. Relax your arm and start again.

Your goal: 3 sets of 10 repetitions

Watch out for: As with the Front Wall Walking exercise, please don't
  hold the top position.

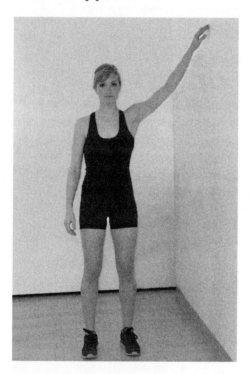

Standing side wall walking

Arm across the Chest Stretch

This stretch is basically done by putting your arm in front of your body
  in the direction we call *horizontal adduction*. This is a real good
  stretch for some who have been told that the tendinitis in their rotator cuff is partly due to posterior shoulder capsule tightness. Opening or loosening up the back part of the shoulder capsule will allow
  the humerus bone to slide back into its natural position and give you
  more range of motion and less pain.

Place your affected arm across your body and put your opposite hand on just above the elbow of the affected arm. Now lightly press your elbow to your chest until you feel a good stretch in the back of your affected shoulder. Try holding the position for at least 30 seconds.

Your goal: 3 × 30–60 seconds

Watch out for: Try to not put the arm you are stretching higher than shoulder-level height. You can place your arm a little lower than shoulder height if the shoulder is bothering you.

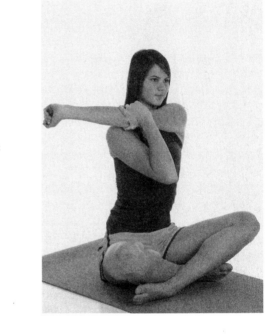

Arm across the chest stretch. *Alan and Vicena Poulson, image from Bigstockphoto.com*

Thoracic Spine Extension Mobility Exercise

This really does wonders for your rib cage area and can help straighten your spine. It looks easy but please move into it slowly. Place your back against the wall, with your lower back flat, causing the lower part of your pelvis to tilt forward. Lift both arms up to 90 degrees. Bend your arms. If at some point you feel some pulling in your rib cage or thoracic spine area, hold the position for 5 seconds and release. If it is not pulling in that position, bend your arms and try

to place them against the wall. Most people feel the stretch at this
point. If you do not, slowly slide your arms up, until you feel a pull
in your spine.

Your goal: 1 set, 5 reps × 5-second hold. You can gradually raise the repetitions to 10 and for 10 seconds when you are able to comfortably.

Watch out for: Your lower back arching. Make sure it is flat against
the wall. Also try to keep your head and arms against the wall when
performing the exercise.

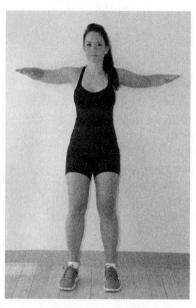

Beginning of thoracic extension
mobility exercise

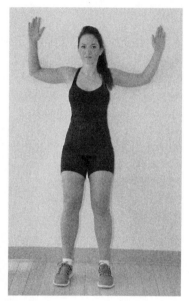

End of thoracic extension mobility
exercise

Latissimus Dorsi Stretch

Here is another great way to get some good range of motion in your
rib cage and to work on your lats flexibility. Start off the same way
that you began you Thoracic Spine Mobility exercise. Place your
lower back flat and head to the wall. Now place the palms of your
hands against the wall. You might start to feel a stretch in the rib
cage region. Hold for 5 seconds if possible, then relax. If you do not

feel pulling yet, slowly slide your palms up the wall as far as you can keeping a proper position.

Your goal: 1 set, 5 reps × 5 second hold, gradually raising it to 10 repetitions and a 10 second hold.

Watch out for: Flaring of the elbows. You might want to let your elbows open up, but try to have them pointed straight ahead, keeping your arms as straight as possible.

Doorway Chest Stretch

This is a very common stretch that will open up the front of your chest area. Don't forget that your chest muscles, along with your lats, are powerful internal rotators and these muscles can give you the appearance of your shoulders' turning inward and giving you that hunched, turned in look. This exercise will help you open yourself up and get you looking straight again.

Stand in the doorway with the arm that you want to stretch placed on the wall with your elbow placed in an "L" position. Next start turning your body away from the door until you start to feel a gentle stretch in your pec muscles and in your front shoulder region. Hold the position for at least 30 seconds.

Your goal: 3 × 30–60 seconds

Watch out for: Try not to lean too far forward with this exercise, as you want to feel the stretch in your pecs rather than a lot of pressure in your shoulder. Also, this should not be done with someone who has an anterior shoulder subluxation, and especially those recovering from a dislocation, as this exercise will only worsen the condition. Make sure that your forearm always stays in contact with the wall and keep your elbow at a 90-degree position when you are doing this stretch. I prefer that you do this stretch one arm at a time versus both arms, as you can really control the movement with one arm and not hurt yourself.

YOUR STRENGTHENING EXERCISES

Even a small change in your rotator cuff strength can make a big difference in the healing of your shoulder, especially if you have lost some muscle due to muscular atrophy. Here are a series of specific strengthening exercises that I believe will really help your rotator cuff get the strength and stability it needs. Strong muscles can help keep your shoulder stable and eventually more comfortable.

Keep in mind that on days that your shoulder might be experiencing some pain and discomfort, you can always either decrease the number of exercises performed or stop the exercises altogether. Also, make sure you are not holding your breath during these exercises. Try to breathe as normally as you can. Holding your breath during the exercises can cause a change in blood pressure. This can cause a problem, especially for people suffering from cardiovascular issues.

Make sure you respect the speed with which you move your weights. Resist jerking or thrusting your weights into the proper position. This might cause a discomfort or injury that you are not looking for. You should try using smooth, steady movements throughout the range.

Do not be surprised that you might be sore the next day. Muscle soreness can last up to a couple of days and slight tiredness or fatigue is really normal after some muscle and strength-building exercises. Keep in mind that none of these exercises should cause you pain. The range in which you are moving your arm and shoulder should never hurt.

There are some exercises that don't require you to move your arm at all. They are called *isometric* exercises. These exercises are different from the exercises that involve movement, as when you lift your arm up and down. Those are called *isotonic* exercises.

An isometric exercise is when the length of your muscle stays the same even if it is contracting. It is done through a static position, rather than being dynamic like the isotonic exercises. The feeling of an isometric exercise is what you get when you are pushing against an immovable object. You will feel a maximum contraction of your muscles, especially your shoulders, but you haven't moved. It has been shown in many randomized controlled studies that isometric exercises can actually improve your strength and make your muscles bigger![2]

Although they are introduced in no particular order, I have put together for you a rotator cuff routine that you can follow. I must reiterate here that you should make sure your doctor has assessed your problem and has indeed stated that you have a rotator cuff problem before attempting the program. This program will do your shoulder problem a world of good!

Isometric External Rotation

I mostly find that my patients' external rotation movement is the weakest of all of the movements in the shoulder. This is due to our daily, bad habits of having our shoulders turn in. It could be that a bad postural sitting position is mostly training the bigger muscles like the pecs and lat muscles and forgetting about the small ones. This is a good starting exercise to strengthen you rotator cuff muscles.

Stand in front of the open doorway with the back of the hand of the shoulder that you want to work on against the doorframe. Your elbow should be at a 90-degree angle. Try to push strongly with the back of your hand against the doorframe for 3 seconds and relax.

Your goal: 3 × 10

Watch out for: Make sure that you face forward when performing this exercise and that your elbow is at 90 degrees. The tendency might be that you want to push it. Push strongly with your hand against the doorframe, but the shoulder has to be as comfortable as possible. Don't hurt yourself.

Isometric Shoulder Flexion

This will start to build the muscles in the front of your shoulder—without the pain. Stand in front of a wall, about 5 inches away. Make a fist with your hand and raise your arm until it touches the wall. Push hard against the wall for 3 seconds and relax. Relax for about 5 seconds in between each repetition.

Your goal: 3 × 10

Watch out for: Make sure you are not twisting your body and that you really feel your muscles working in the front of your shoulder.

Isometric Shoulder Abduction

This exercise is the same as the isometric shoulder flexion, except you will be pushing to your side instead of to your front. Stand sideways to the wall, again about 5 inches or so away. Making a fist with your hand, and raise your arm until it touches the wall. Push hard against the wall for 3 seconds and relax. Try to rest for about 5 seconds in between each repetition.

Your goal: 3 × 10

Watch out for: You will get a better contraction if you push with your wrist instead of just your hand. Also try not to shrug your shoulders or tilt your trunk.

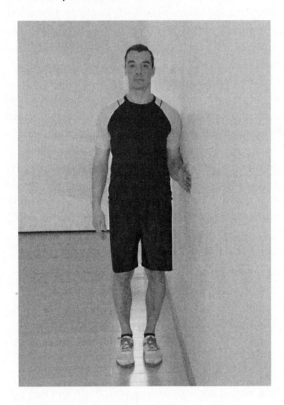

Isometric shoulder abduction

Side Lying External Rotation

This exercise will really strengthen the external rotators of your shoulder, which are almost all your rotator cuff muscles, and save your subscapularis muscle. Lying down on the side opposite your injured shoulder (e.g., if your right shoulder is injured, then lie on your left side), stick your elbow to your side. Place a folded towel or a small pillow between your elbow and your body. Bend your arm at a 90-degree angle and rest your affected arm on your rib cage. Make a fist. Your knuckles should be facing the floor. Now keeping your wrist straight, lift your fist up and back as high as possible and pointing to the ceiling. The movement should be done pretty quickly—in approximately 1 second or so. Don't worry if you can't do this in the beginning. It will come with practice. Hold that position for 2 seconds, and then slowly lower the arm for a count of 3 seconds.

The speed of your exercise should approximately be: 1 second up, 2 seconds hold, 3 seconds down or 1–2–3. Always start with no weight in your hand and try to complete 1 set of 10 repetitions. If you find that simple, then try the next set with one pound, and so on, until you can do the exercise with a 5-pound weight. This might not be as easy as it looks, so don't be surprised that you can't perform the movement as easily as you thought.

Your goal: 3 × 10. Rest 30 seconds between each set.

Watch out for:

1. *Wrist*: Keep it straight (i.e., in line with the forearm) at all times. If the wrist bends, then the movement will come from the forearm and not the shoulder. Try to think that your wrists are hooks and can't turn. Also ease up on your grip. It makes a world of difference!
2. *Elbow*: Sometimes the elbow might slip forward as you are performing the exercise. Keep it stuck to your side!
3. *Back*: Try not to rotate backward toward the floor as you are lifting the weight.
4. *Neck*: Make sure your head is resting comfortably, with no tension in your neck when you lie sideways. Use two pillows if you have to.

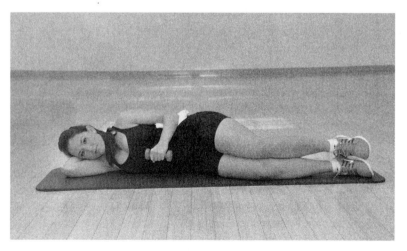

Beginning position of side lying external rotation

Visualize: You are lifting the weight with your shoulder, and not the forearm. You might feel a burning down the outside of your arm. Eventually you will feel it in the back of your shoulder.

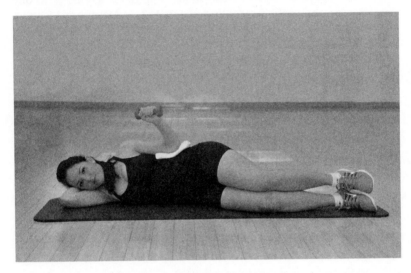

End postition of side lying external rotation

Side Lying Lifting Arm Straight Up

Lie down again on the side opposite to your injured shoulder, with your arm in front and perpendicular to your body. Make sure you start the position with your arm resting on the side, or as low as you can go. Keeping your wrist straight, lift your arms to the ceiling quickly, again in approximately 1 second, hold the position for about 2 seconds, and lower all the way down in 3 seconds. Try not to rest the arm completely, but stop a couple of inches from touching the bed. This puts continuous tension on your muscles, which will make them work even harder.

Your goal: 3 × 10. Again, start with no weight, and increase the weight by one pound, until you can lift 5–7 pounds for the 3 sets. Try to rest for 30 seconds in between each set.

Watch out for: Make sure your arm is at 90-degrees to your body, not higher. If your shoulder is uncomfortable in this position, lower your arm slightly toward your feet, and try the exercise in that position.

Visualize: You are lifting the weight up with your shoulder, and not with your forearm. Ease up on the grip when holding the weight. You should not feel the tension in your forearm. You should feel some contraction in your upper shoulder blade, in the back of the shoulder or arm. That's a good thing!!

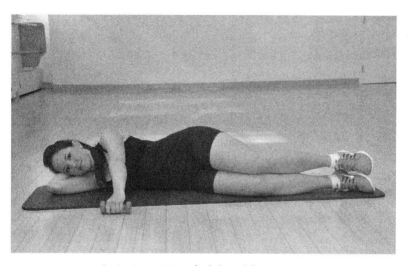

Beginning position of side lying lifting arm up

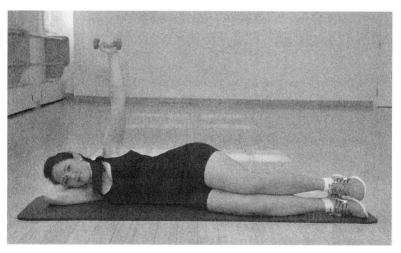

End position of side lying lifting arm up

Side Lying Alphabet

Now here is a fun one! You will stick out your arm in front of you and make a fist as you did with Side Lying, Lifting Arm Straight Up. This time, however, instead of moving up and down, you will draw the letters of the alphabet! (I have trouble sometimes remembering all the letters, too!) Always write small letters and not capital ones. In addition, try to make them as large as possible with your arm still in front of you. If you have to stop at some point during the exercise because your muscles feel like they are on fire, then stop. Take a break, catch your breath, and once you are good and ready, continue until you finish the alphabet. It might take some time to increase your endurance and that is okay. Your shoulder has not been put through endurance training for a while and it is adjusting. Be patient and keep trying!

This will build strength in your shoulder, as well as increase your endurance.

Your goal: 1 × alphabet. Try to get from *a* to *z* without stopping!

Watch out for: Not bending your elbow or wrist at all through these movements. Your arm should be kept straight, with the work coming from the shoulder. As always, make sure your neck is comfortable.

Shoulder Blade Push-Up

This is a great exercise to strengthen your serratus anterior muscle, which helps with stabilizing your shoulder blades. Get into a push-up position. If the position is really challenging then it is okay to try it on your knees instead of up on your toes. Try to keep a nice, straight line from the top of your head all the way down to your feet. While you are up in the push-up position, try to contract the muscle that brings your shoulder blades together. Hold for 2 seconds then return to the original push-up position

Your goal: 3 × 10

Watch out for: If you are arching your back, try to keep a straight line. Also try to have your weight over your fingers and the whole hand, not just the heel of your hand. You will gain better control of the movement if you use your whole hand.

Airplane

This exercise really works on the muscles in your shoulder and upper back, and all the muscles in between. This exercise is named *Airplane* because if it is done properly, you will look like an airplane! Lying on your stomach, bring your shoulder blades together and bring your head slightly back, lifting from the floor; turn your hands outward so that your thumbs point to the ceiling. Hold the position for 10 seconds. Eventually, you will progress to doing this exercise with a 1-lb. weight in each hand, and will try to increase it to 5 lbs.

Your goal: 1 × 10. Each repetition: 10 seconds holding the position and 10 seconds resting between each repetition.

Watch out for: The way you rotate your arms. A way to know if you are performing the exercise correctly is to bring your shoulder blades together. In one way, you will be able to bring the shoulder blades really close together; the other way will move them further apart. Use the way that moves your shoulder blades closer together.

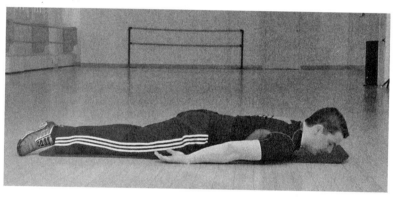

Beginning position of airplane exercise

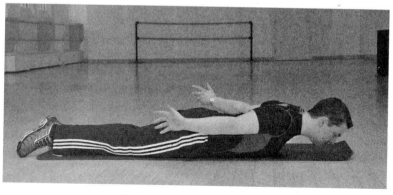

End position of airplane exercise

Superman

This will really work on bringing your shoulders back, opening you up and making you look straight and tall again, instead of the hunched-over posture position that most of us develop at work. It is one of the best scapular stabilizing exercises that you can do anywhere. It is named *Superman* because you will look like you are flying!

Start by lying on your stomach; bring your arms toward your head, shoulder width apart. Point your thumbs to the ceiling. In this position, try to lift your arms as high up as you can, keeping them there for a count of 10 seconds. You could then bring them down and relax for 10 seconds. Eventually, you will progress to doing this exercise with a 1-lb.weight in each hand, trying to increase the weight by one pound each time, to eventually reach the 5-lbs. level.

Your goal: 1 × 10. Each repetition: 10 seconds holding the arms up and 10 seconds resting between each repetition.

Watch out for: If you find it too hard to lift your arms up in the position that you are using, bring your arms further away from your head, until you can lift your arms up and hold the position. The closer your arms are to your head, the harder it is. Only when your arms are almost touching your head should you start with 1-lb. weights or move up in weight.

If you like, you can also do this exercise with one arm, but I prefer that you start with two arms to balance out both of your sides.

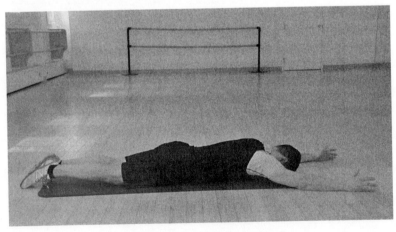

Beginning position of superman exercise

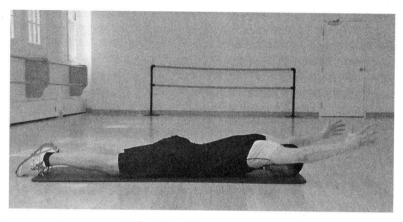

End position of superman exercise

Shoulder Raise in Sitting

In a sitting position, lift your arm up to the ceiling, with your arm in front of you, in 1 second. Hold for 2 seconds, and slowly lower your arm for a count of 3 seconds. Make sure the arm stops just before the position it can rest in. You want the arm to be working continuously.

Your goal: 3 × 10. Start with no weight, and increase the weight until you can lift 5 lbs. for the 3 sets without any real problems. Rest 30 seconds in between each set.

Watch out for: If you can't lift your arm all the way up, it might be due to the lack of range of motion (ROM) that you need but don't have. Please then refer to the ROM exercises section of

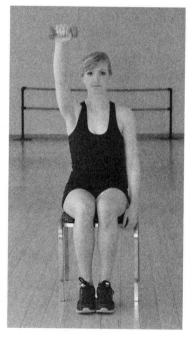

Shoulder raise in sitting

the book. Make sure you get full ROM first, or else you will become stronger in the range that you have, and that's it.

Forward Alphabet in Sitting

Start in the same position as the above exercise, Shoulder Raises in Sitting, but this time, keeping your arm in front of you, try drawing the alphabet from *a* to *z* without stopping (unless you need a break, of course!) with your hand in a clenched fist.

Your goal: 1 × alphabet without stopping. Start with no weight, eventually moving up to 5 lbs.

Watch out for: When performing this exercise, try to keep your arm up above 90 degrees of flexion. That is, don't drop your arm down to your side, but keep it higher than having your arm in front of you. Try to maintain a good posture position and try to make your letters as big as possible, using the largest amount of space in front of you to draw your letters. As with the previous alphabet exercise, if you get tired, please take a break, catch your breath, and continue.

Arm to Your Side in Sitting

Start in a sitting position with your arm hanging at your side, palm facing your body. Lift your arm up to your head in 1 second. Make sure your arm is still at the side of your body and not in front of you. Try to hold the position for 2 seconds, and then lower (deliberately) in 3 seconds. When you hold the position for 2 seconds, make sure you are not resting. You always want continual tension placed on the muscle that you are trying to work on.

Your goal: 3 × 10. Start with no weight, and increase the weight by 1 lb. until you can lift up to 5 lbs. to your side for 3 sets with no problems. Rest for 30 seconds in between each set.

Watch out for: When you are lifting your arm, make sure it is to your side, and not coming forward. If your arm is coming forward, it might be that the weight is too heavy for you. Decrease the weight by 1 lb. and continue. If the sitting position is too uncomfortable for you, you can always try it in a standing position.

Alphabet with Your Arm at Side in Sitting

Begin in the same position as the previous exercise, so that your arm is perpendicular to your body and try to write the letters of the alphabet from *a* to *z* without stopping. Try to write the letters in lower case and not in capital letters.

Your goal: 1 × alphabet without stopping, preferably moving up from no weight, to a 5-lbs. weight.

Watch out for: When writing the alphabet, try to not drop your arm too low, but stay in the 90-degree range and above. You should really feel the burn in your shoulder, but not a sharp stabbing pain that makes you want to stop immediately. Also, if the weight is too heavy for you, you will start to bring your arm forward. Try to keep the weight to your side as much as you can or lower the weight.

Please know that this is not a complete list of every shoulder rehabilitation exercise known. There are countless others, done with different methods and techniques, which will give the same results. A lot of these exercises can be done with elastic bands, tubes, canes, and all sorts or other apparatus. My belief is that you can use any method that you like as long as you feel what you are supposed to be stretching or strengthening, and that it is not painful but feels good. The exercises and programs below are the ones that I have chosen and recommend to you and I hope that they will help give you some relief.

ROTATOR CUFF ROUTINES

Levels 1 and 2 go together, as do levels 3 and 4, and levels 5 and 6. Level 1, 3 and 5 should be done on Monday, Wednesday and Friday and levels 2, 4, 6 should be done on Tuesday and Thursday. Saturday and Sunday should be the days that you give your shoulders a break and let them get stronger and looser.

It is a very good idea to place some ice on the front of your shoulder, until frozen, after your workout. This will reduce the irritation caused by the exercises, and it will provide you with soothing relief.

Level 1 Exercises

1. Supine Stick Flexion: 2 × 10
2. Bent Over Arm Swings and Circles, or Pendulum: 2 × 10
3. Arm across the Chest Stretch: 2 × 1 minute
4. Isometric Shoulder Flexion: 2 × 10
5. Isometric External Rotation: 2 × 10

Level 2 Exercises

1. Shoulder Blade Push-Up: 2×10
2. Doorway Chest Stretch: 2×1 min
3. Standing Front Wall Walking: 2×10
4. Standing Side Wall Walking: 2×10
5. Side Lying External Rotation: 2×10

Level 3 Exercises

1. Supine Stick Flexion: 2×10
2. Standing Front Wall Walking: 2×10
3. Standing Side Wall Walking: 2×10
4. Side Lying External Rotation: 2×10
5. Side Lying Lifting Arm Straight Up: 2×10
6. Side Lying Alphabet: 1×1 alphabet

Level 4 Exercises

1. Thoracic Spine Extension Mobility: 1×5 (5 second hold/rep)
2. Latissimus Dorsi Stretch: 1×5 (5 second hold/rep)
3. Side Lying External Rotation: 2×10
4. Side Lying Alphabet: 1×1 alphabet
5. Airplane: 1×10

Level 5 Exercises

1. Thoracic Spine Extension Mobility: 1×10 (10 second hold/rep)
2. Latissimus Dorsi Stretch: 1×10 (10 second hold/rep)
3. Airplane: 1×10
4. Sitting Flexion: 2×10
5. Sitting Abduction: 2×10

Level 6 Exercises

1. Superman: 1×10
2. Airplane: 1×10
3. Sitting Flexion: 2×10
4. Sitting Flexion with Alphabet: 1×1 alphabet
5. Sitting Abduction with Alphabet: 1×1 alphabet

Hopefully, these exercises will really help your shoulder get strong and supple enough to help you return to your sport, activity, or just daily life. If these exercises are not really helping your condition, make sure you see your doctor, physiotherapist, or any allied health professional.

CHAPTER FOUR SUMMARY

- A 20-minute warm-up prepares the muscles, heart, and nervous system, and is a hedge against injury.
- The eccentric phase of an exercise repetition is as important as the concentric phase and should be given equal attention if you are to achieve the kind of balance that can keep injury at bay.
- The 3 × 10 formula for an exercise routine—three sets of ten repetitions—boosts endurance and strength effectively and safely.

5

Fix Your Posture, Too

"I want to get old gracefully. I want to have good posture, I want to be healthy and be an example to my children."

—Sting

Good thinking on Sting's part: Posture and health are inextricably linked, far more than most people realize. Sure, we've all felt that "crick" in the back of the neck that makes us almost mindlessly stretch upward and press our shoulder blades together.

Ever find yourself slouched in your chair at work, not realizing why your shoulders ache or why you feel a spasm in your upper trap muscles? No, it is not because you are old; it's because your horrible posture is causing you anguish and pain! Without good posture, you can't really be physically fit.

WHAT DOES IT MEAN TO HAVE A GOOD POSTURE?

Having a good posture means that you maintain an ideal spine throughout your body. And having an ideal, natural spine really means to achieve the three natural curves that keep your spine healthy and happy for a long life.

The three natural curves are in the cervical, thoracic and lumbar regions. You might also have heard (especially for all you Pilates fanatics) about a "neutral pelvis." This means trying to get the top of your pelvic bone (commonly called your ASIS or the anterior superior iliac spine of your pelvis) in a vertical plane with your pubic symphysis, which is an area made of cartilage that separate your left hip or pubic bone from your right hip or pubic bone.

A therapist looking at your posture looks to see if you deviate or fall out from the middle or plumb line. We look at you from the front, side, and back to see if your head is too far forward, if your shoulders turn in, and if your pelvis tilted—along with a host of other things. We examine you from your head down to your feet for anything that might look different from the normal.

It is important to know that proper posture should be maintained while sitting, standing, and sleeping.

Why should we maintain a good posture? The whole point of having good posture, other than the obvious one of not getting injured, is to try to keep the proper position of the body's different parts so that the least amount of energy is required to maintain a position that you want. This position, if achieved, places the least amount of stress on the body's tissues. Good posture also has been shown to improve breathing greatly and minimizes negative effects on the body's fluids doing their jobs. As people admire your amazing posture, whether standing or sitting, you will also get a lot of positive looks coming your way, almost in the same way people gawk at someone who is in shape and walks proudly because of it!

OKAY, WHAT DOES IT REALLY MEAN TO HAVE POOR POSTURE?

What poor posture really means is that your body has developed muscle imbalances due to your daily activities and habits. Some of your muscles shorten or tighten up, while other muscles stretch out and are lengthened, giving you no support at all. Repetitive movements and other biomechanical factors, such as different forces placed on your body, can create postural problems. It has been also shown that workers with a higher stress level are more prone to develop neck and shoulder symptoms.

Poor posture can contribute to chest pain. This is because we may sit in a hunched or slouched position at our desk during the day. Our lungs can't fully expand and our shoulders start to turn inward, causing pectoral muscles to tighten up. We start taking less and less deep breaths and chest pain starts to develop. Large-breasted women seem to develop this problem of hunching and rotating their shoulders inward.

I personally believe that strengthening the muscles in the back area of your shoulder blades and other stabilizing muscles that we will talk about in the forthcoming chapters will alleviate that hunching position. This increases your capacity to breathe and balances out the strength and flexibility of your front and your back.

It is very rare to see some with a very strong upper and lower back with a very weak front. As humans, we tend to look at and train the areas of our body that we see on a daily basis. We normally look at the front of our body, and want to make it look better and stronger. We forget the back part of our body, because basically, we don't look at it as much. If we trained and took care of the back part of us as much as we did the front part of us, we would have fewer postural issues, and definitely less pain and discomfort.

Most, but not all, posture-related problems, come from sitting. As a society, we watch more television than any other previous generation. We drive more and we fly more now than in the past—often in poorly designed seats. A lot of us work in sedentary jobs day after day, or work in front of computers. If you are not in an ideal postural position, then daily improper repetitive positions can wreak havoc with your body. Some of the other factors that can contribute to poor posture can come from excessive weight, a mattress or pillow that is not right for you and gives poor sleep support, improper shoes, careless sitting or standing habits (I am guilty of this one as well), a poorly designed workspace, and as stated before, occupational stress.

THE FORWARD HEAD POSTURE

Did you know that your head on your spine weighs approximately 12 pounds?

According to Kapandji, "for every inch of forward head posture, it can increase the weight of the head on the spine by an additional 10 pounds."[1] It is not uncommon for a patient to come into the clinic with a head that has moved from one to three inches forward from the shoulders. That can come out to 42 pounds that your posterior neck muscles have to try to hold up all day, every day! Eventually, these muscles throw in the towel and call it a day. The way they do that is by sending you a pain signal to stop you from holding that position when your head leans in too much to see the computer screen.

When the head is that far forward and adds 42 pounds of additional leverage and pull on the cervical spine (neck region), it can possibly pull the spine out of normal alignment. According to Dr. Rene Caillet, MD, a forward head posture can result in a loss of 30 percent of someone's vital lung capacity due to the loss of the cervical lordosis (the natural curvature of the neck).[2] By decreasing the cervical lordosis, this forward head posture limits the hyoid muscle's action to lift the first rib when inhaling. The gastrointestinal region, especially the large intestine, becomes irritated from the forward neck posture that can cause sluggish bowel function and execution. This is pretty serious things to consider. Dr. Caillet advises people to work on their head position before working on the body, because the body will follow the head, but not necessarily the other way around.

When our head is forward in this bad postural position for a long period of time we can develop something called *Upper Crossed Syndrome*. First talked about by the famed biomedical researcher Dr. Vladimir Janda, this syndrome is created by tightness and weakness in the levator scapula and your upper traps, the suboccipital neck muscles, the sternocleidomastoid muscles of the neck, and the pectoralis major and minor. On the opposite side you have lengthened or overstretched muscles of the rhomboids major and minor, the middle and lower trapezius, the serratus anterior, and the deep anterior neck muscles. Due to the fact that the patient has stayed in this bad position for days, months, or even years, the body has developed new nerve pathways for this position and made it the "new normal."

If you start to change head and neck positions quickly, it will make the wrong muscles work instead of the right ones; the secondary muscles will try to do the work of the primary ones and everything will be out of whack. It has been said that the best way around this is to try to loosen up those stiff dysfunctional joints in your neck, to try to loosen and hopefully reprogram those nerve pathways. Once we see that those joints are moving properly, we can start working on muscles tendons and other soft tissue to recreate the balance of strength and flexibility that is needed.

By improving your upper body posture, your shoulder blades will come closer together and not allow the stretching and subsequent weakening of the rhomboids or the middle and lower trapezius, which can no longer firmly anchor the shoulder blades to your more stable thoracic spine. These muscles, in addition to their own specific functions, act on transmitting forces from the daily activities of lifting, pushing/pulling weight from the arms to the bigger spinal column of your back. If these muscles become strong and healthy, they will stabilize the shoulder blades, and very little force will go to the more delicate neck region through the upper traps and levator scapulae muscle—even if you lift something heavy.

Some of the traits seen in someone who possibly has an Upper Crossed Syndrome are:

- Difficulty swallowing
- Clenched teeth
- Mouth breathing, which causes sleep apnea
- Migraine headaches
- Severe neck pain

THORACIC OUTLET SYNDROME

Thoracic outlet syndrome or TOS is a rare, painful condition that can come from depressed shoulders. Symptoms may include waking up from your sleep with tingling or numbness in your hands, as well as weakness in your arms and hands. This normally can happen due to a compression of your brachial plexus, which are a collection of nerves that works the sensation and motor function of your entire arm, from the side of your neck to your fingertips. This compression can come from a depressed clavicle or collarbone, which decreases the space in the shoulder—a space that is already particularly small—and can lead to numbness and tingling caused by compression of the brachial plexus.

But there is no need to worry. Your physical therapist or allied health professional can help you with this condition.

You can achieve great posture by training your body to stay in positions that put less strain on your supportive muscles, ligaments, and joints. Proper posture can also decrease some of the wear and tear on your joint surfaces, possibly reducing the potential for osteoarthritis.

One technique that can help right away is to have a higher awareness of your posture at all times. Practice makes perfect! If you practice this "new and improved" posture for standing and sitting on a consistent basis, it will gradually replace your old posture.

Unfortunately, when you have bad posture, such as a slouched sitting position, the weight distribution of your body becomes unbalanced: you put too much pressure on certain areas, such as your neck and shoulders, and not enough on other areas, resulting in grief and discomfort.

Improper posture can also prevent the appropriate muscles and ligaments from working properly. This will cause compression (impingement) of the shoulder muscles, due to the fact that the shoulder blades are turning in too much and causing your upper back to curve out. This creates an altered and stressful change in the position of your shoulder in relation to the rest of your body, and potentially leads to a rotator cuff injury.

PROPER POSITIONING

Let me take a moment to explain where the ideal position for the scapula should be. All too often, your scapulas abduct or fan outward to the front of the body and rotate upward. Ideally, they should be adducting or coming to the spine and rotating downward. To achieve this position, you need to strengthen the rhomboids and mid and lower trap muscles, which will help pull the scapulas together as well as pull them down. We will go through those exercises in chapters that follow.

Poor posture also increases neck pain and stiffness (due to the fact that your head is leaning too far forward with respect to the rest of your body). This occurs when you want to massage those muscles to get rid of the pain and discomfort. But if you can correct your posture, your problems will disappear, and you will feel a whole lot better (not to mention people will notice you and comment on your amazing posture).

If your excessively forward head and turned-in shoulders consistently stay in that position for lengthy periods of time, without being corrected, you will eventually have increased difficulty performing certain everyday functional movements—for example, combing or blow drying your hair, putting your shirt on, putting dishes away, lifting heavy grocery bags, and so forth.

How do you know that the pain that you are getting is due to your bad sitting or standing posture position?

The following are some of the telltale signs that you might feel:

- Getting tension across your upper back and between the shoulder blades
- Feeling spasms on your upper neck (you know you have experienced this feeling if you performed a couple of circles with your head today, just to get rid of the spasm)
- Numbness starting from your neck down to your arms (possibly contributed to by your less-than-ideal sitting position)

- Experiencing constant headaches, starting at the bottom of your skull
- Feeling consistent and recurring upper trap spasms. This is a very common sign. You are always pressing down with your thumb or fingers on your upper trap area to get it to stop contracting so much!
- Experiencing difficulty in swallowing
- Hearing cracking noises as you move your head about
- Not understanding why you always bring your shoulder blades together during the day
- Performing continuous backward shoulder circles
- Getting up almost every hour to walk around or go to the bathroom (People will think that you are healthy, because you are always drinking water!) Although it is very easy to say this comes from stress (blame it on your boss), it really comes from the way you are sitting in your chair at your desk or in front of the computer.

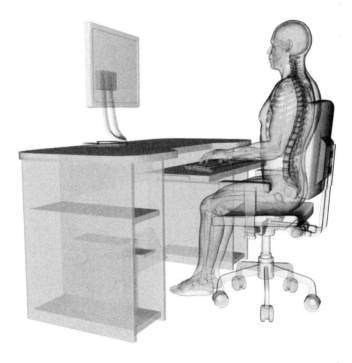

Proper sitting posture. *Sebastien Kaulitzki/Shutterstock*

MUSCLE SPASMS

I think this is one of the great mysteries of our time (up there with the flying baby stork and the secret to the Cadbury chocolate bar): Why do we get muscle spasms?

For example, let's take the muscles in the back of your neck. You sit in your chair in a slumped position. (You are not doing that now because we all know that you are sitting up straight.)

If your head is leaning forward, gravity is trying to pull your head to the ground. But the muscles on your neck are trying to pull your head back.

It's the classic tug-of-war.

Who will win? Gravity will never stop pulling. After a short while, the muscles in your neck will start to get tired from trying to pull your head up. What else can they do? They will go into a spasm to protect them-selves from overstretching.

Unfortunately, that's when your brain says, "Oh, not another neck spasm!!" You instinctively start stretching out your muscles for that in-stant relief. And you will get the relief, but it will be temporary. The cycle will then begin again with the muscles on the back of the neck, not being strong enough to keep your head up, going back into spasm.

Therefore, the reason that your muscles go into spasms is that they are weak—not that they are tight.

So what does one do? Should you call in sick, lying in bed and thinking that the end of the road is near? Should you compare horror stories with your friends, so that you completely freak out?

The best thing to do to help yourself is to look at the way you are sitting.

Creating a good workstation position is very important to your health. You can improve your position at your desk at work or at your home by trying some of the following helpful hints.

DYNAMIC SITTING

Try not to sit in the same position for long periods of time. I suggest get-ting up and walking around every hour. Stretch out, pet your dog, or do something that will get you out of that same, static position.

Look at the position of your chair. Your chair should have some kind of back support. It is not necessary to buy an expensive or state-of-the-art chair, just as long as there is a small cushion to support your lower back. Having support in your lower back will help take the strain off your neck and will bring your shoulders back, keeping them in the more ideal position.

If you don't have any professional lower back support—for example, a lumbar roll—then a small pillow or even rolled up towels will do the trick. Whatever you use, make sure it is placed in your low back, just above the belt level of your pants or in the small of your back.

The height of the chair is also important. The chair should be high enough so that your feet rest flat on the floor.

Check that your knees are at a 90-degree angle to the floor.

Don't forget to look at the position of your mouse and keyboard. They should be close to your body. Ideally, with your arms tucked to your side at 90 degrees, the mouse is in your right/left hand or very close to it. Also, your keyboard should be at your fingers' reach with your elbows at 90 degrees. If you constantly reach forward, you can possibly get shoulder pain that radiates down your arm, as well as a neck spasm.

Another area to look out for is cradling the telephone between your shoulder and neck so that you can talk while you work on your computer. This is a recipe for disaster! Keeping the phone in this position will cause neck spasms, shoulder pain, and headaches. We definitely don't want that.

You know that something is wrong when you sit at the edge of your chair. Make sure you sit all the way back, or have your knees resting 1–3 inches from the edge of the seat. You should adjust your armrests so that your elbows are 90-degree angles while typing.

YOUR COMPUTER MONITOR SCREEN

Your monitor should be one arm's length away from your head.

The height at the top of the screen, or at least the top third of it, should be at the same level as your eyes. Also make a fist with your arm extended in front of you. The computer screen should be touching your fist. If it is further away than that, you might be leaning too far forward in your chair. If the screen is lower, you will have to look down, pulling your head forward and causing your neck muscles to go into a muscular spasm.

Also, make sure you place your computer or home monitor parallel to your windows to minimize the glare that you might get from the sun, or at least use an antiglare screen.

CHECKLIST FOR OPTIMUM SEATED
POSTURE POSITION

- *Neck*: Neutral; pay attention so your head does not come or tilt forward
- *Shoulders*: Neutral; avoid slouching or leaning forward
- *Upper arms*: 90 degree angle and close to your body
- *Hands*: In line with your forearms, wrists neutral
- *Back*: Leaning on lumbar roll with lower back, keep spine with its natural curves, try to keep your pelvis in a neutral position. If you find yourself sitting at the edge of the chair, that might mean that your chair is just too high up and you are trying to come lower down. Try lowering the seat so that your torso is all the way back touching the back of the chair.
- *Thighs*: Knees should be approximately at 90 degrees and thighs parallel to the floor
- *Feet*: Flat on the floor

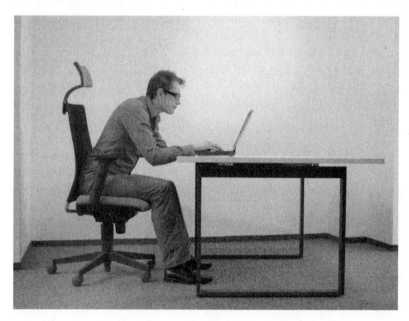

Man in improper sitting posture. *Narcin Balcerzak/Shutterstock*

STANDING POSTURE

To have the proper standing posture does not mean to just stand up straight. There are a couple of pointers that I will give you that if followed, can really help you with your posture and reduce those aches and pains that you might be experiencing.

If you want to feel what a proper upright position should really feel like, stand against the wall, with your back on it. Do you find yourself leaning forward and bending at your mid-back? If you are not sure, try taking a deep breath in. Do you find yourself lifting yourself upward, lifting your chest up, decreasing the excessive kyphotic curvature in your thoracic spine and making you feel better? Once you start noticing the bad habits that you have been doing unconsciously, you start to win the battle. Most people don't know at all or have very little consciousness of what is the right posture.

WHAT ABOUT YOUR LOWER BODY?

Please pay close attention to your feet. Do you find that you are putting weight on the soles of your feet equally or on one foot more than the other one? Also, please look to see that you are not putting a lot of the pressure on the ball of the foot and big toe. If you are, it means that you are probably leaning forward. If you are experiencing back pain, this might be a contributor. Try to keep your body evenly placed between your heels and the balls of your feet.

Look at your knees. Are they hyperextending? Try to bend them a bit, but not flex them too much. If you are not sure how to correct it, then seek a medical professional to help. When you are bending over, try to bend at the hips and not from your back (which will round your back and place a strain on it). When your back is rounded, you are most prone to injuring yourself.

Leaning forward places a considerable amount of force and strain on the back part of you, sometimes called the *posterior chain* of your body. This consists of the posterior muscles of the trunk and your legs, which remain in constant contraction. They try, every day, to pull you up from your forward position, so that you don't fall forward and land on the floor. Your tight hamstrings try to bring your pelvis backward. (Poke your hamstrings now. Do they feel tight?) And your pelvis tries to tilt backward to pull your lumbar spine and the rest of your body up. You can only imagine how exhausting this might be for your muscles.

We all try to work so hard and so fast that we don't realize what we are doing to ourselves—and that becomes a bad habit. Bad habits can happen from sitting, standing, or even running, and they become very hard to break but they can be reversed.

Some individuals don't believe that they can change their posture. They will say that they are old and have accepted their fate, or that their parents have bad posture and, because of genetics, it will happen to them. Sometimes when I look at a patient, after they have told me about their shoulder or neck injury, I might respond by stating that their bad posture might be a reason for their condition. Looking shocked, they might respond by saying that people have said that they have great posture or personally always believed that they have great posture. They look at me as if I am nuts! Only when I bring them in front of a mirror and show them their body, explaining to them where the body should be positioned, do they start to understand.

Sometimes people don't think that their muscles are weak and can stay weak. They think that the muscles will get stronger naturally. The famous quote, "If you don't use it, you will lose it," applies here. It is almost like an elastic band that people tie their hair with. It might be strong in the beginning, but if you keep pulling on it, day after day, it starts to stretch out. In the beginning it might be strong enough to hold the hair in place, but eventually it will loosen up and stay loose. Once it is too loose, it no longer works to do its job anymore, so we throw it away.

Muscles that become overstretched and looser kind of work the same way, except for the fact that we can't through them away. We need to strengthen them, getting them tighter and creating the right balance in the area so we can function optimally. Don't think that just because we put in all that work to get those muscles stronger and working great and to maximum capacity, we can go back to our bad postural habits. If we do, then the aches and pains will come back again for sure.

I believe that it is a choice a person must make if they honestly want to preserve the most valuable thing that they have: their own body.

CAN GOOD POSTURE ACTUALLY GIVE YOU POWER?

According to a study done by Carney et al.,[3] "posing in high-power nonverbal displays" for example, sitting and standing properly and tall actually creates chemical changes to the body. The people who are "high-power posers" and have great posture have increased level of testosterone, decreases in the stress hormone cortisol, and increased feelings of power and risk appetite. However, for someone who is slouching, or in this study someone who has a submissive closed posture, the opposite effects are shown. Bottom line: If you want to really feel better, work on that posture and look up, instead of closing yourself in and looking down.

WHAT DOES AN IDEAL POSTURE REALLY LOOK LIKE?

If you drew a line straight down your body when you stood sideways, the following would be the ideal position for that line to pass through:

- Slightly in front of your lateral malleolus, or the outside bump of your ankle,
- Slightly in front of the middle of your knee joint,
- Slightly behind the middle of your hip joint,
- Going through the bodies of your lumbar vertebrae or low back,
- Through the tip of your shoulder joint,
- Through the bodies of your cervical vertebrae or neck area,
- Through the middle part of your earlobe, specifically the external auditory meatus,
- And lastly, through the mastoid process of your jaw.

The following are different types of faulty posture: the flat back posture, the swayback posture, and the kyphotic-lordotic posture.

The Flat Back

A flat back posture really means what it implies: Your low back, called your *lumbar spine*, is completely straight, instead of having the necessary lordotic curve that it needs to absorb stress and impact. This normally happens because the pelvis is turned under (a posterior tilt). This straightening can also have a negative effect on the thoracic region by decreasing the curve there and making the head lean forward. In a nutshell the body would look like this: Head too far forward, neck or cervical curve increased, the shoulders leaning forward and downward, the chest falling forward, upper and lower back straightened out, the pelvis turning backward, and knees tending to be hyperextended or locked. The tight muscles will be the abs, hamstrings, and the front and side neck muscles. The spine will be pretty stiff as well.

Keep in mind that you do not need to show every characteristic of a flat back to be suffering from many of the symptoms associated with it. Some individuals, according to the research, show a very strong posture type but show no symptoms, while others complain and suffer greatly from minimal posture problems. Every case is different.

So how can we fix this? The best place to start is always the center of the body, at the pelvis. Increasing mobility and trying to adopt a more neutral pelvis position is a good first step. Next, work on stretching and loosening of the hamstrings, as well as strengthening the abdominals. Work on your obliques instead of just your rectus abdominis, and your spine will thank you. Work on the strengthening of your hip flexors, called your *iliopsoas* muscles. This will work to increase the curve in your lumbar spine, but don't forget to strengthen your lower back muscles, which will further help increase that curve. Your physiotherapist or allied health professional can help you with that.

Your upper back should be also loosened up and its tension decreased as much as possible.

The core solution to this issue, therefore, is to get your pelvis aligned to neutral, but also try to figure out why it became tilted that way. Most times it comes from your sitting position at work. A proper sitting position should feel like you are sitting on the top of your legs, and not feeling like you are placing your entire weight on your buttocks muscles.

Areas to strengthen: Your psoas major and minor, as well as your iliacus muscle. These muscles make up the iliopsoas muscles and are commonly referred to as the *hip flexors*.

Areas to stretch: primarily the hamstrings.

The Swayback

The swayback posture is very different from the flat back posture. Whereas in the flat back posture, your lumbar spine has no curvature, in the swayback position, the opposite is true. The swayback individual has an excessive curvature of the lower back. This position can place an abnormal, uneven amount of stress on the discs and joints in the lumbar spine. A swayback position is seen more commonly when the person is standing up, rather than in a sitting position. It is more commonly seen in women than men, especially when wearing high heels. High heels can cause the pelvis to tilt forward and contribute to the swayback. Another reason that women would have more of a swayback than men is due to the bigger "padding" in the gluteal or buttock region.

People with swayback have really tight hip flexors that can also be caused by daily sitting for very long periods of time, which will eventually turn that movement into a bad habit. The solution to this postural problem, again, is to try to get the pelvis back to its natural, neutral position. A good way to stretch your hip flexors and strengthen your abdominal muscles is by doing the Plank exercise, which helps maintain the pelvis and spine in a more neutral position. The Plank, an oldie but a goodie, works all the different layers on the abdominals. Another beginner exercise that is given is call the Pelvic Tilt exercise, which can really help out a swayback and can relieve a lot of your lower back pain.

Your therapist would probably make you go through a specific analysis of your posture. This might include looking at your alignment from your head, neck, shoulder, and spine, all the way down to your toes and in every direction. They will also put you through some special tests designed to measure your muscle strength and the areas where you are mostly weak. Lastly, they will look at your range of motion and the stability of your joints, as well as the flexibility of your muscles. Based on all this information, they will then come up with a comprehensive exercise program for you. Your therapist will go through it with you to see if you are doing everything properly, so you will not injure yourself.

Areas to strengthen: One-joint hip flexors, the external oblique abdominals, your upper back extensors, and the muscles that flex the neck.

Areas to stretch: Hamstrings and the lower back region as well as the internal obliques. Your therapist or your health professional can help you with this.

Kyphotic-Lordotic Back

This is a posture where all the curves become greatly exaggerated.

Starting at the neck, the curve becomes exaggerated, as in a hyperextension position, which brings the head greatly forward in comparison to the sternum. The upper back or thoracic spine becomes curved (like a hunchback), creating an increased thoracic kyphosis, and the shoulders are rounded forward. The lower back also has an exaggerated curve, creating a hyperlordotic curve, thus creating a pelvis that looks tipped, called an *anteriorly tipped* pelvis. This posture is common and frequent in individuals who I have seen.

This posture can lead to back pain, irritations of nerves, up to causing some heart problems. It is therefore imperative to correct this postural problem. As in the other two postures that we have seen, some muscles are overextended and weak, which would need us to get them stronger, and other areas are shortened and need to be stretched out. It is always about achieving the correct balance.

In this type of posture, the muscles that are overstretched and weak are as follows: the neck flexors, the erectus spinae muscles (a deep muscle layer found in your back), the transverse abdominis muscle (the deepest abdominal muscle in the body), and your hamstring muscles. The muscles that are normally found to be very short, tight, and too strong would be the muscle extensors of your neck, like the trapezius; your pectoral muscles; and the flexors of the hip, your iliopsoas muscles as well as the rectus femoris muscle of your quadriceps.

Areas to strengthen: Hamstrings, glutes, and your transverse and oblique abdominal muscles.

Areas to stretch: Hip flexors, rectus femoris, pecs, and lower back.

Handedness Posture

When I ask questions in my history taking, there is always one question that gets a quizzical look from patients: Which is your dominant hand? But it is important to know when you are looking at posture and the risk of musculoskeletal injuries. Here is how Kendall describes the posture of someone with a dominant right hand, or right-handedness posture.[4]

Lengthened and weak:

Left sided trunk muscles
Right hip abductors
Left hip adductors
Right peroneus longus and peroneus brevis
Right tensor fascia latae
Left posterior tibialis
Left flexor hallucus longus/digitorum longus

Shortened and tight:

Right-side trunk muscles
Left hip abductors
Right hip adductor
Left peroneus longus and brevis
Left tensor fascia latae
Right posterior tibialis
Right flexor hallucus longus
Right flexor digitorum longus

Again, according to Kendall, when you look at the posture of the client with a right-handed posture, you will probably see a right shoulder that is lower than the left, a lateral pelvic tilt with the right hip joint adducted and medially rotated, and some pronation of the right foot.

Did you know that 30 percent of the population are lefties and hold their pen or writing implement differently than the right-handed people? Lefties place their wrist in an over-flexed position, and with that comes a bigger risk to developing carpal tunnel syndrome than the rest of the population.[5]

Lower Cross Body Syndrome

In 1987, the great Dr. Vladimir Janda, a true pioneer in muscle imbalances, described a lower cross body syndrome (LCS), otherwise known as the *pelvic crossed syndrome.* This is caused by a tightness of the thoracolumbar extensors on the back, which cross with the tightness in the iliopsoas and rectus femoris muscle of the quadriceps. The weak, deep abdominals cross with the weak gluteus maximus and gluteus medius muscles. This cross pattern of imbalanced muscles causes havoc at the joints creating dysfunctions at spinal segments L4–L5 and L5–S1, as well as at the sacrum itself and the hip joints.

Posture changes that you can see with this dysfunction include your pelvis tilted forward, an increase lordosis on your lumbar spine, a lateral shift of the low back, lateral leg rotation, and the knee hyperextended.

One must also look at the lordosis: If it is short and deep, it probably means that the imbalance is with the pelvic muscles, but if it goes all the way up to the thoracic region and looks shallow, then it probably implies that the imbalance is at the trunk or abdominal muscles.

Layer Syndrome

This syndrome, sometimes referred to as the *stratification syndrome*, is really a combination of the upper cross syndrome and the lower cross syndrome. Patients with this problem have lived with it for a long time and their inability to regulate their motor control, would lead to a poorer prognosis than if the patient just had an upper or lower body syndrome by itself. This condition is seen in older patients and patients with unsuccessful disc surgery. Some of the imbalances you see with a layer syndrome include:

Weakness: Lower stabilizers of the scapula, lumbosacral erector spinae, and gluteus maximus.

Tightness: Cervical erector spinae muscles, upper trapezius, levator scapulae, as well as the thoracolumbar erector spinae and hamstrings.

WHAT CAN WE DO ABOUT THIS PROBLEM IN THE MEAN TIME?

You can try using two full-length mirrors to see yourself from the front and from the side. Although you won't be able to look at yourself from the back, I think you can still collect some valuable information about what you are doing wrong, and start adjusting yourself to attain a better posture. This exercise will start to work on your proprioception and body sense, which is half of the battle. If you realize, for example, that your shoulders are turning in and hunched forward, you might start practicing to bring your shoulders back. Doing it repeatedly will help your awareness until one day, with all the exercises that you are doing to help, your shoulders will stay back.

You can also have someone take a picture of you lifting something or videotaping you doing something that you do on an everyday basis, and then you can take a look and analyze yourself. Do not be surprised if what you actually see on the tape is not what you thought you were doing.

Even though bad posture is not hereditary, bad postural habits or tendencies for bad habits might actually run in the family. Take a look at your family members when they are sitting watching TV or at the dinner table. I am sure you will see some common habits that they themselves don't realize that they are doing. Do they have a swayback or a flat back, or do you maybe see a fit person who has a ton of energy and looks pretty good. That might be someone you might try to emulate.

Don't get me wrong, no one is perfect. I am not perfect either. Tired from working, I got a flat back, which limited my pelvic flexibility. I didn't realize how my pelvis really was until one of my therapists told me about it. I wasn't experiencing any back pain, but I knew that I would have to nip this problem quickly if I didn't want any issues later. I strengthened the appropriate areas and immediately felt a positive difference.

ABDOMINAL CRUNCHES

Why are crunches bad for your posture? I thought that they were good for me!

Modified sit-ups like trunk curls or crunches have been a staple in peoples' exercise routines for a very long time. Here is why you are advised not to work on them. Continuous and repeated work on your rectus abdominis muscle, a band of muscle that runs from your rib cage to your pelvis, will weaken your external obliques, which really need to be strengthened to prevent having both a swayback and a kyphotic-lordotic back.

Think of a crunch movement. When do we really do that movement on a daily basis? Rarely. The oblique muscles, however, are responsible for one important movement: turning or rotation. We twist and turn all the time, yet though my experience, I have seen that people would rather do crunches than those rotational exercises. Obliques are also important because of their stabilizing contribution to the trunk and pelvic regions.

Another reason that repetitive flexing exercises are not ideal is that they can cause continual lower back flexion, which can stress the lower back and produce pain. This type of exercise should be avoided by women who are postmenopausal due to their risk of osteoporosis and compression fractures of the spine.

I SEE THAT MY HEAD IS FORWARD RELATIVE TO MY BODY. WHAT CAN I DO ABOUT IT?

As we stated earlier, for every inch your head goes forward there is an extra 10-pound weight placed on your neck. Many people are surprised to learn that they have bad neck posture, so here is a little test that you can do to see if your posture is the reason you are not in an optimal position.

After you determine that you need to have your posture corrected you will need to stretch and strengthen certain muscles with appropriate exercises.

Here is what you should do:

Stand up with your back against the wall. Put your feet at shoulder width apart and try to get your shoulder blades to touch the wall. A good tip is, by slightly bringing your shoulder blades together, try to get them (rather than the top of your shoulders) to touch the wall . You should not try to get the top of the shoulder blades to the wall because you will overcompensate by arching your back. This could lead to more pain and discomfort.

Now please check to see if the back of your head touches the wall or not. Don't worry if it doesn't. It is not as easy as it sounds. First try to bring the back of your head as far back as possible, making it touch the wall.

Next, try this image: Visualize a long piece of thread or string coming out of the top of your head, and pull that string to the ceiling. It is going to create an image of your neck being longer. As the back of your neck starts to get longer, you might find yourself doing a chin tuck or developing a second chin. If you are, you are doing it correctly. Just be careful that instead of making a chin tuck you are not just moving your head backward, because it is not the right way.

Try thinking of making the neck as long as possible, or as if someone is trying to pull your head to the ceiling. What you are trying to accomplish is called *traction*. Hold this chin tuck position for about 1 minute maximum. If you can't or it hurts, try this method: Instead of holding the position try doing something called *chin retractions* or *frequent chin tucks* from the amazing people at the Robin McKenzie Institute.

You can do this from sitting up, but if you prefer lying down on your back, that might just work more easily for you. Lying down on your back with your knees bent, look at the ceiling with your nose approximately perpendicular to the ceiling. Try either the double chin technique, or alternatively, try nodding your head slowly without your neck moving. Try keeping the movement slow so that you can really feel the stretch in the back of your neck. If you feel a bit of tension in the front, don't worry as long as you are feeling more tension in the back of your neck—as if the vertebras and muscles are pulling apart.

In this exercise, you are not really holding it at all but doing the movement frequently. The count would be: chin tuck one second, relax for one second, then repeat. My suggestion is to try for 10 chin retraction repetitions per hour. In theory, this method should be done, but if it is not possible to do it that many times, then try to perform the exercise as frequently as possible throughout the day.

It is possible that you might feel the pull starting in your neck and moving down to your shoulder blades. That is okay. Please don't overpush or overstrain yourself. Try the motion just enough to get a pulling sensation and eventually that pulling will turn into a release sensation. Once you really get used to the movement and the feel, you can then practice it up against the wall or anywhere you want. Your end goal is to be able to push your chin in to the fullest and without getting any pulling in your neck at all, and with no discomfort.

Next, let's work on your shoulder blades.

Sitting in a chair with your knees bent 90 degrees and your neck nice and long, practice just dropping your shoulders down. This sounds easy, but many people have so much tension built up in their traps that they can't put their shoulder blades down. All these exercises take practice and patience to get them right.

Try squeezing your shoulder blades together, as if you are trying to crash them into each other. Hold this position for 3–5 seconds, then release to the beginning position. Try performing this exercise daily for 3 sets of 10 times with good muscle control. Do not be surprised to see that it is actually harder to control the release of the contraction to the shoulder blades' beginning position, than actually doing the contracting. A slow, controlled release is called an *eccentric* movement. When the hold of 3–5 seconds becomes easy, you can increase to a 10-second hold. Try doing this exercise daily, if possible.

The end goal for this exercise is that you can get your rhomboid and other rib cage/shoulder stabilizing muscles to start working and developing muscle strength. It will also help to naturally raise your chest. It is hard to keep your head up and in its ideal position if your shoulders are droopy and sagging forward. If you notice during the day that your shoulders are in front of your chest, doing this exercise will really set the shoulder blades into their right place.

MATTRESSES AND SLEEPING

Getting a good night's rest is really important for good health. Therefore a good mattress can really help with your posture and help with any shoulder or any other pain that you might be experiencing.

To start with, I am a believer that your mattress should be a firm one. What do I mean by that? A firm mattress should be able to give slightly when you lie on it and should feel a little stronger than other plusher or softer mattresses. This is not a set rule, just a guideline if you don't know where to start looking. Your mattress choice will depend upon you and what your body feels right.

If a mattress is way too hard, then it won't really support your body evenly and there will be some unnecessary pressure points that you won't really be able to relieve or get rid of. This will make you toss and turn all night and not really give you that restful sleep that you are looking for.

However, you also don't want a mattress that is so soft that you sink into the bed, because that will throw your spine, shoulders, and the rest of your body off its proper alignment. This will make your muscles keep working throughout the night to make them align the spine, with little success. A strong movement—turning around quickly for example— might just pull your muscles enough to give you aches and pains when you wake up. How many of you experience a neck ache or *torticollis* when you wake up, and you are stiff and sore for the rest of the day? I know that it happens really often.

The most important thing to do is to go to a mattress store and lie down on the first bed you see. I don't think the sales representative would mind. In fact I am sure they will encourage you to keep trying their mattresses until you find the one that is right for you.

If you would like a mattress with a long life, then the type of upholstery materials as well as the type of steel that is used to create the mattress is important. Also, if you plan to do your homework on this mattress, consider if the springs found inside the mattress recoil back to their original position or not. Also, try to find a mattress with the largest number of springs possible, and ask if they will maintain their shape over time or not. That will greatly affect their durability. Mattresses are not cheap, so try to go with the one that will give you the best comfort at the right price.

Please do not forget to look and test the mattress's box spring, found underneath the mattress. The box spring is supposed to increase the length and longevity of the sleep system. It does this by absorbing a big part of the weight that is placed on the sleep surface—kind of like a shock absorber—so that the mattress can last longer. The more steel added in the box spring, the more durable it becomes.

There are a lot of different mattresses out there, so give them a test drive!

WHAT IS A POSTURE BRA?

A posture bra claims to do what its name implies: It is a bra that will help a woman's posture. It can do this by helping support the upper back and relieve pain, headaches, and possible long-lasting dysfunctions in the person's thoracic spine. This will really help with someone in a crouched position in front of a computer all day. A posture bra will buy you some strength, support, and endurance that you need to get through your days. This support will also reduce the stress that you normally feel because of muscle weakness in your back.

Although this might feel great, I would suggest that in the mean time, you really start to strengthen your back muscles so that you do not need to wear this support bra forever. It is really temporary until you get stronger. You don't want it to become a crutch.

A great thing about the back support or posture bra is that it can teach you the proper position that your spine should be in, kind of a form of biofeedback. Once the body starts to learn and understand the correct position that it is supposed to maintain, the position will be easier for the individual to hold and maintain it. The faulty position will decrease and the bad habits that you developed at work will start to change.

Posture bras have been carefully constructed with material that is comfortable and gives enough stretch that it will give you a nice fit. Some stronger materials strategically are also placed to give you that support in your thoracic spine. Other bras can also provide you with support in your lower back and in front of your chest, giving additional support to the breasts from the front and from the sides.

The most important thing to look for in one of these types of bras is the best fit for you. Make sure that all the straps can be adjusted, even the strap in the back. See if the shoulder straps are adjustable, if they can be changed for an occasion, from color to invisible. Some companies that make these bras are called *EquiFit* and *Exquisite*.

Although posture braces are not talked about here at length, they can help an individual with a severe postural problem. As with the bra, they should be used temporarily, until the strength and endurance come back in the muscles. Your doctor, physiotherapist, or other professional might give you one to help with your condition.

Here are some other little tidbits to keep in mind:

- Never carry heavy bags, purses, or backpacks if possible. Do not carry backpacks or heavy bags on one shoulder because that can lead to improper posture alignment, leading to discomfort and pain.
- Try getting up from your computer or TV and walk around once every half an hour so that moving around decreases some of the pressure in your neck and shoulder.
- If you have difficulty sleeping or wake up with a sore neck or shoulder, try using a supportive pillow. With a strong curved section located at the bottom of the pillow, these pillows let your head fall into the middle of the cushion, giving your neck nice support.

I really wanted to give you a slight overview in the sitting and standing positions, and get you to start practicing them.

Taking care of your posture is not that difficult, but the benefits can be amazing! (You might even get some positive comments from your friends and family.) All you need to do is to go over these general points at the place that you are sitting, and you body will thank you so much.

6

For Workout Warriors, Moves to Avoid—Or at Least Modify

"A man's gotta know his limitations."

—Clint Eastwood

When I was a teenager, I was hell-bent on getting big and strong. I thought having strong, sculpted muscles in all the right places was a way to impress important people and garner compliments on my fitness. I also felt pretty sure it wouldn't hurt my chances with members of the opposite sex.

My problem was that I also needed to keep up with my schoolwork and maintain my grades. That did not give me a lot of time to train. I needed to get to the gym, perform my workout, and get out of the gym as quickly as possible. As for so many people today with full lives and hectic schedules, time was of the essence for me.

So I tried to follow other people's routines, giving little thought to what I was really doing. At the time, I wasn't too concerned about what the speed of an exercise movement might have to do with anything, and concentrating on performing the exercise correctly and efficiently was also of little importance. I just wanted to do my gym routine and go back to enjoying my life with my friends.

Sound familiar? Ever find yourself in a hurry because you had an appointment later but decided you really, really needed to get in a quick workout first? So your aim was to finish the workout as quickly as possible, get out of the gym, and get on with your life. To do so, maybe you just copied the exercises you saw someone else doing, or you remembered that quick routine you read about somewhere in some magazine and just did whatever it is you remembered.

Fair enough—except that while some exercises are really good for you and can make you stronger and leaner, they still have to be done properly. At the same time, there are some exercises that not only won't really help you, but can also create or exacerbate a shoulder injury. You certainly don't want to squander valuable gym time on movements like that.

So if you have any type of shoulder injury—and certainly if you have been formally diagnosed with a rotator cuff problem—I suggest you refrain from doing some exercises altogether. Now, you're probably asking yourself why I would devote a whole chapter to exercises you should *not* do if you want to avoid shoulder problems and shoulder pain. Basically, there are two reasons:

First, I think it's important to understand why and how these exercises may be harmful. I know that many of you are, if not gym rats or fitness freaks per se, certainly concerned about your physical well-being and committed to getting and staying in the best condition possible. I believe that the more you know and understand about how the body works, the better equipped you will be to address your concern and carry out your commitment.

Second, I know too that many of you will be very reluctant to give up, even temporarily, the kinds of benefits you're accustomed to getting from these exercises, a number of which are standards and favorites among even casual gym goers. So I want to offer you, in addition to an understanding of the harm you may do to yourselves, some workarounds and modifications for performing the exercises so that you can gain the exercise benefits you seek without risk—and certainly without pain. I suggest, however, if these exercises are part of your normal routine, or if they help you fulfill other physical goals, that you please check with your professional health practitioner about doing the modified exercises I offer. He or she should be able to advise you as to whether even these modifications might exacerbate your particular situation. Better safe than sorry, and above all, you don't want to do yourself any real harm.

Here are the exercises to watch out for if you have shoulder problems or a diagnosed shoulder injury:

Chest Dip
Chest Stretch
Chest Fly (starting from low on the body)
Barbell Behind-the-Neck
Upright Row
Lat Pull-Down Behind the Neck
Dumbbell Bench Press (starting low on the body)
Neck Bench Press
Supraspinatus Fly
Push-Up

CHEST DIP

The Chest Dip is normally performed on a specialized exercise-dipping machine or between two parallel bars. The point of the exercise, effected by lowering yourself below the bars, is to work the lower chest muscles, the front of the shoulder, and the triceps muscles, thereby toning your arms, chest, upper back, and shoulders. But because the exercise affects the shoulder directly, if you already have a rotator cuff injury, unfortunately the exercise can place a lot of extra stress on the front part of your shoulder joint.

The issue is primarily a matter of your position with respect to the bar. If your upper body leans too far forward or your shoulder tilts too far back, your position produces an upward and forward force to the shoulder blade, and causes a painful impingement to your rotator cuff region. And typically, if you're suffering shoulder pain or have a shoulder injury, the tendency in doing the Chest Dip is to allow the shoulders to rise up toward the ears or to fall back as if the shoulder blades were being squeezed. Also typically, people trying to get the most out of the Chest Dip bounce off the bottom and this can place even more unnecessary stress on the shoulder joint. In a word, the deeper into the movement you go, the worse the stress on the acromioclavicular (A/C) joint of the shoulder. Remember the A/C joint from chapter 1? One of the four major shoulder joints, it both connects the shoulder to the rest of your body and is what enables your arm to enjoy full range of motion. Done incorrectly, Chest Dips can damage the acromioclavicular ligament, the main ligament of the shoulder joint, potentially causing an A/C separation, which can take a very long time to heal.

Is there a way to keep the Chest Dip in your program so that you avoid exacerbating a shoulder injury or adding to your pain? Let me put it this way: There are certainly some precautions you can take so you don't get hurt. In fact, these precautions are useful any time you perform a Chest Dip, whether you have an injury or not; they will help keep you free of injury so that you can get the most out of this exercise without endangering your shoulder.

First of all, *warm up*. Of course, it can't be stated too often that you should always warm up before starting any form of exercise, but I also know that we all sometimes forget to do so. The best way to warm up if you're concerned about your shoulder is with a light shoulder routine. The isometric exercises described in chapter 4 are good examples to follow. Alternatively, even a chest exercise routine using really light weights will work, but be sure to use truly light weights—ones you can use for approximately 15–20 repetitions. Remember that the purpose of the warm-up is to get your shoulder ready for the routine, not to power though the movement.

A second caution is to be sure you *control the eccentric or negative part of the movement*. In the Chest Dip, that is the downward dip, as opposed to the upward movement. Failure to control the downward dip results in a quick fall, which stresses the shoulder, so be sure to keep your mind on what you're doing and stay in control of that downward dip. Your shoulder will thank you.

Third, be sure *not to go too deep* in the movement. Yes, the point of the Chest Dip is to get a really good stretch, but this can be dangerous. It is best not to let your elbows bend more than 90 degrees—that is, don't let your upper arm go past being parallel to the floor. Doing so will strain the shoulder and make you worse, rather than better.

Fourth, *breathe right*. That means you should inhale on the downward dip, exhale when you come up.

Fifth, watch the *placement of your hands*. Placing your hands far apart will work more chest fibers, but placing the hands too far apart can place a strain on the shoulder. Keeping the hands close together produces more triceps contraction in addition to the Chest Stretch, while resulting in much less chest and shoulder pain.

Finally, go *easy on the weight*. We all want to fight greater resistance when it comes to Chest Dips, so it is very tempting to go for heavier weights. Don't do it. Only after you are comfortable doing more than

12 reps with a light weight should you even consider adding weight. Even then, increase the weight by just a couple of pounds, but not more than that.

By the way, you can get a similar stretching and contraction effect on the chest with a decline dumbbell press—without affecting the problem shoulder.

CHEST STRETCH

The pectoral or Chest Stretch is justifiably renowned for opening up the chest and helping to balance the upper torso. I see people doing the Chest Stretch in the gym every day, and a lot of them tell me they do it because they have shoulder issues. Some say they have been advised to do this stretch because they have "rounded shoulders." Yet "rounded shoulders" may be a big contributor to rotator cuff syndrome, and I, for one, certainly would not self-stretch my chest muscles if I had that kind of shoulder pain or injury.

Why not? If you start off with a shoulder rotator cuff injury, and you do a further stretch, you are "opening" up the back end of the glenohumeral (G/H) capsule, the envelope of ligaments that surround the ball-and-socket shoulder joint. That can cause the head of the joint to slide forward, and that, in turn, can cause an impingement shoulder syndrome injury—and can hurt like crazy.

There's a much better way to get the same toning and balancing effect—without threatening your shoulder joint and risking the pain and discomfort of a shoulder injury. It's to strengthen the rhomboid muscles connecting the scapula to the spine, and at the same time to work the lower trapezius muscles in your upper back where they converge with the scapula. Strengthening the rhomboids by bringing your shoulder blades together will naturally open the shoulder area in the front of the body, will reduce compression on the long head of the biceps tendon, and will help rectify any imbalance of strength between the front and the back of the shoulder region. Strengthening the lower traps, which tend to be overstretched and weak from overactive upper trap activity—and from bad upper back posture—will retract and depress the scapula, unrounding your rounded shoulders and helping to make your torso balanced, strong, and very aligned.

CHEST FLY (STARTING FROM LOW ON THE BODY)

Chest Flys are another exercise that, if you are not careful, will overstretch the front part of your shoulder capsule and injure the rotator cuff. The function of your pectoral muscles is basically to bring your arms together toward the center of your body, and that is what you do when you perform this exercise—except that you are using weights, cables, or in some cases, an exercise ball. The problem with doing flys is that, even though you are on your back, the arc of your movement needs to be tightly controlled. Extending your arms too far back or going too far down toward the floor can affect your shoulders. This effect is worse if your arms straighten; your arms should always remain bent. The effect is still worse if the weight used is too heavy.

My advice is to stop doing flys altogether till your injury has completely healed or your shoulder problems have totally disappeared. But if you insist on doing them, use light weights and lower them only to the level of your body—no lower. Yes, you are trying to get a stretch in your pecs when coming down, but if you go down too low, you will do yourself much more harm than good.

An alternative way to perform your Chest Flys is on a seated fly machine. On such a machine, you can preadjust the setting so that the pads come down only to your sides. This gives you the pump you need without the injury.

BARBELL BEHIND-THE-NECK PRESS

Lifting a barbell overhead behind your neck is an exercise aimed at developing the front and side deltoid muscles of the shoulder, the shoulder's "lifting" muscles, as well as the upper traps. It is a common exercise, yet as far as shoulder health is concerned, I personally believe that it is one of the most dangerous exercises you can do, risking a rotator cuff injury with every press. Just think about it. Every time you bring the weight down, you force the elbows forward and the hands backward, and this really works the shoulders.

The issue is rotator cuff flexibility. In the starting position of the press, you need full external rotation of your shoulders while they are abducted at 90 degrees; your upper arms are parallel to the floor, while your fists holding the weight are pointing to the ceiling. The next phase of the movement requires bringing the shoulder blades slightly together; this is shoulder retraction. If you cannot comfortably and fully do either of these movements, chances are you lack the necessary flexibility for this exercise. That means that if you do the exercise anyway, you will almost surely injure yourself.

What impact does this exercise have on the structure of the shoulder? The internal rotators—the pectoral and latissimus dorsi muscles—get too tight, and this tightness increases the pressure and strain on the external rotators, primarily the infraspinatus and teres minor muscles. Added weight exacerbates that pressure and strain. The more weight you hold, the worse the pressure and strain. The tiny muscles of the external rotators become overburdened, and the result is a mechanical breakdown of the rotator cuff region, biceps tendon, or other structures. Simply put, something gives way.

The Behind-the-Neck Press can also affect the neck region. If you do not have adequate shoulder external rotation, you might try to compensate somewhere on your spine, either by excessively rounding your upper back or by doing something or other to move your head and neck forward. Don't forget that your upper traps contract very hard during this exercise, and if your neck is not stable or strong, a neck strain could result. Also, any forward head position will stretch the neck, adding to the stress and very possibly causing a neck injury.

So the risks associated with Behind-the-Neck Barbell Presses are, in my view, far greater than any benefits to be gained—especially because there are so many other exercises you can do to strengthen your shoulders, as we'll see in chapter 7.

If you have to do Behind-the-Neck Presses, at least do them with dumbbells. You need better coordination and more control with dumbbells than with barbells, so use a lighter weight until you get the proper lifting form down pat. Of course, doing barbell pressure in front of the body, starting at the upper chest area and lifting upward, provides the same strengthening benefit as the behind-the-neck movement, but places no pressure on the rotator cuff or other muscles.

UPRIGHT ROW

The Upright Row calls for an overhand grip on the weights or barbell and lifting the load from waist level up to the collarbone. It is an exercise many people rely on to build up their shoulders, upper back and upper traps. The problem comes from doing this exercise if you have bad posture to begin with, as do so many people who sit at a desk all day. This means you are starting off the exercise with your shoulder blade tilted upward and sticking out. This puts your shoulder into too much internal rotation, and a set of Upright Row exercises will only further decrease your shoulder's flexibility. You'll just be in the wrong position to do Upright Rows effectively.

Even if you have been doing Upright Rows without any problem for some time, you are still at risk of developing a shoulder impingement syndrome. Once the syndrome starts, it is just a matter of time before the shoulder becomes so inflamed and painful that you are unable to do anything, much less work out.

Again, I do not recommend this exercise for anyone with shoulder problems, shoulder pain, or a weak shoulder, but here are some tips to help those who insist on doing it. First, try to develop your lower traps, which tilt your shoulder blades backward. Strengthening the lower traps will counteract the forward rotated position that the Upright Row develops in the upper traps. Also, take great care not to stick out your neck when you do the upright lift or you risk severe neck pain and headaches. Raise the weight until your upper arm is at an angle of 90 degrees to your body, no higher. Anything greater than a 90-degree angle puts the shoulders into internal rotation, very dangerous for rotator cuff problems because it forces the arms inward, too, and subjects the shoulders to enormous and unnecessary stress.

Keep the weight light and avoid a swinging motion when raising it. Technique in the movement is particularly important for reducing stress on the shoulders, so focus on a straight-up lift—no thrusting or lurching. And be sure you have a controlled grip.

Better yet, spend your time on other, more pertinent, less dangerous exercises.

LAT PULL-DOWNS BEHIND THE NECK

Pulling a weighted cable down behind the neck in order to strengthen the broad latissimus dorsi muscle of the back presents many of the same issues as the Behind-the-Neck Press. In fact, you tend to relax the shoulder while performing a pulldown, and you're likely to bring the bar down really low in an attempt to gain that elusive "extra" stretch. But the fact is that the pulldown, while especially dangerous for someone with rotator cuff problems, will adversely affect anyone with any kind of shoulder issues.

Lat Pull-Downs stress the front of the shoulder joint, causing strain at least and possible injuries at worst. They also stretch a network of nerves, called the *brachial plexus*, which extend through the neck, thereby creating a tingling or numbness in your arms. Pushing the head forward to get it out of the way of the downward bar leads to pain and discomfort in the neck or shoulder, and in most cases in both, especially if the individual is using too much weight.

Again, the same strengthening can be achieved more easily and equally efficiently by pulling the bar down in front of the body—to about the level of your upper chest.

DUMBBELL BENCH PRESS
(STARTING FROM LOW ON THE BODY)

In general, exercises done with dumbbells are preferable to those done with a barbell. They are gentler on the shoulders and enable better individual control of the movement. But sometimes, even with dumbbells, overzealous individuals going for that maximum stretch on their pecs will take the weight so low as to stress the front part of the shoulder excessively, risking injury. This typically happens when the individual does the presses while holding the arms much too close to the body; that's what drags the weight down too low.

To avoid that, either use a barbell, or be very careful to lower the weight only until the elbows are parallel to the shoulders and extended slightly away from the body. Either way offers the same stretch effect to the pectoral muscles.

NECK BENCH PRESS

The Neck Bench Press, also called the *guillotine press*, was originally developed and recommended by the "Iron Guru," legendary bodybuilder Vince Gironda, back in the 1950s. Although it has been shown to yield good results when it comes to strengthening and sculpting the chest, this exercise can make a weak shoulder even worse, so if you have any kind of shoulder problem whatsoever, be assured that the risks of the Neck Bench Press outweigh its benefits. You're lying back, holding the weight in a fairly wide grip, starting the lift from just above the neck, and returning the weight to neck level. In doing so, your shoulders are flared out to the side instead of close-in to the body as in a regular bench press. Yes, this may achieve better pectoral stimulation, but it also affects the back of your shoulder joint, where you are likely to feel a sharp, sudden pain. The reason is that as you lower the weight to your neck, your arms are wide apart and away from your body, effecting a shearing or pulling action that opens up your shoulder joint.

A simple modification to the exercise can help—namely, bringing the bar down to your lower chest rather than to your neck. This puts your arms in a more natural, shoulder-width position and thus greatly reduces the stress on your rotator cuff and shoulder.

Again, other bench press exercises avoid the possible adverse impacts of the Neck Bench Press altogether.

SUPRASPINATUS FLY

A Supraspinatus Fly, also known as the Empty-Can Fly, was developed by Dr. Frank Jobe, a well-known shoulder specialist. It is normally performed like a front shoulder raise, but at a 45-degree angle. You hold a very light weight—or an empty can—in front of you with your thumb lower than your pinkie, as if you were pouring water. You then lift your arm up until it is at a level that is about 60 degrees of flexion or, where the aim is to isolate the supraspinatus tendon, all the way up toward the ceiling.

This exercise is incorporated in a lot of rehabilitation programs as a way to strengthen the rotator cuff, but in fact, it does nothing of the kind. On the contrary: this is a dangerous exercise, for when you raise your arm straight up as far as it can go, you invariably send the shoulder into extreme internal rotation—the very movement you should be trying to avoid. Yes, such a movement may increase the supraspinatus muscle contraction, but it will also cause an impingement injury and can only increase inflammation and pain. In fact, I find the empty can exercise a reliable test for possible impingement problems, and I use it to show me how bad a patient's impingement may be.

One possible workaround for this exercise is to use a full can and hold it with your thumbs pointing up. Electromyogram (EMG) tests of the electrical activity in muscles have shown that the supraspinatus activity in both versions produces the same amount of stimulation. The difference is in the middle deltoid, which gets more stimulation with the empty can. But our purpose is to strengthen the rotator cuff, not stimulate the medial deltoid. Another purpose is to alleviate pain, not cause it; the empty can version of the Supraspinatus Fly hurts, while the version using the full can does not.

Yes, it makes a lot of sense to strengthen the supraspinatus and rotator cuff muscles. There are exercises aimed at doing precisely that; we'll learn all about them in chapter 7 when we set out to create a super shoulder.

PUSH-UPS

"Drop down and gimme 20!" It's a manly cry, and the manly response is to do even more than 20, especially if a woman is watching. But testosterone aside, the Push-Up is an exercise that is likely to exacerbate rotator cuff problems and shoulder pain. Why? Take a look:

The aim of the Push-Up is to get the chest to touch the floor. Yet doing so puts an excessive load on the back of the shoulder capsule and thus stresses the capsule and strains the rotator cuff muscles. Continuing to do the exercise "through" the pain is a pretty certain path to a tendinitis—especially for anyone who has had a previous dislocation or whose shoulder has some looseness or laxity to it.

Remember that one of the major functions of the pectoral and latissimus dorsi muscles is internal rotation of the shoulder. Performing Push-Ups certainly increases internal rotation of the shoulder, but that places tremendous strain on external rotators, which are pretty small compared to your internal rotators and tend to be weak to begin with. This imbalance between the big, strong internal rotators and the small, weak external rotators is the reason some bodybuilders have that turned-in shoulder look. But looks aside, over time imbalance can lead to an impingement of your shoulder.

One way to avoid such impingement is to lower the body until the upper arm is parallel to the floor—that is, the elbows are at a 90-degree angle. Another tip is to place your body weight not on the heel of the hand, as people tend to do, but on the pads of the palms and the pads of the fingers. This actually activates your shoulder blade muscles much more, which in turn can increase your shoulder's stability. It also releases the stress on the capsule and decreases the strain on the rotator cuff.

But the best way to avoid the damage Push-Ups can do is to strengthen your external rotators first. It's all part of giving you a super shoulder that can withstand just about anything, and that's what we'll turn to next.

7

Your Super Shoulder

"Can't I just do cardio for this thing?"

—Robert R., a former patient

Fixing your shoulder is one thing, but it's really only part of the battle. Remember that useful saying, one of many, by America's great revolutionary hero and statesman Benjamin Franklin that "an ounce of prevention is worth a pound of cure"? Now that you've done the hard and maybe lengthy work of the cure, it's time for the prevention program of exercises—strength-building exercises to improve your stability and give you the confidence to do things you once thought you might not ever have the power to do again.

It's pretty simple: You and I both want to make sure you avoid the rehab clinic or the surgeon's scalpel for good as you stay strong, fit, and active. The best way to do that is to get your shoulder into super shape so that you ensure the flexibility and power—and usefulness—of your shoulder muscles for a lifetime.

HOW DO YOU DO THAT?
HOW DO YOU MAKE MUSCLES STRONGER?

The fact of the matter is that the body, which is an amazingly ingenious creation, can adapt extremely well to forces and stresses placed upon it. Maybe you've noticed people working out in the gym for months and months, applying themselves assiduously, yet never seeming to effect any noticeable bodily changes. They look the same after their fiftieth workout as they looked after their first workout. Why? Almost certainly, those people do the same routine comprising the exact same exercises and lift the same amount of weight in every workout they do, workout after workout, week after week, month after month. Well, it pretty much stands to reason that if you keep doing the same thing, you'll get the same result. If you change nothing, you won't see any change in your body or any change in your level of strength. Why should you?

The secret is the body's efficiency. It will do what is demanded of it, but nothing more; that is how it conserves the energy it needs to power you through your day—and through your life. So if you do one set of Front Dumbbell Raises with 15-pound weights for months on end, your body "understands" it need only be strong enough to lift 15 pounds—not an ounce more. That is its point of stability, and it will stay at that strength level until a greater force or stiffer demand is made upon it. There's even a name for this expression of bodily efficiency and stability; it is called the *General Adaptation Syndrome.* Simply put, the body has adapted to the exercise demands placed on it to the point that, as far as your muscles are concerned, no change is needed.

So what do you do to gain strength in your body? It's simple: You give your muscles a reason to raise the level of their efficiency and stability. I like to think of it as a process of shock and awe: You change some element in your exercise routine, introducing a behavior or practice your body is not used to, and this so surprises the muscles that it jolts them into a responsive action. You were using 15-pound dumbbells for Front Dumbbell Raises? Try 20-pound dumbbells. You were accustomed to doing 3 sets of 8 reps? Try 3 sets of 10 reps, or maybe 5 sets of 8. You used to rest for one minute between sets? Try limiting your rest to 30 seconds, and see what happens.

For one thing, in each case, you feel the difference. Accustomed to a 15-pound dumbbell, your body suddenly struggles to lift 20 pounds. Your muscles simply weren't ready for that change. Remember they had adapted to 15 pounds, so they are shocked at this new demand being made on them and awed that it's for a full 5 pounds. They need to readapt. And that's exactly what they do. During the rest time you give your body, the cells of the muscles (their tissue and fibers), and the energy centers of the muscles will expand to meet the demand placed on them by the new weight. Keep it up, and over time, the muscles adapt upward to the new standard you have set.

The same thing happens if you increase the number of sets or reduce the length of your rest breaks, even if you're still lifting 15 pounds. Increasing the number of sets requires more endurance; taking shorter rest breaks makes it tougher on the body to recover. Both actions make it harder to lift the same weight again, and the new demands stimulate your muscles to get stronger for the next time.

Of course, the reverse is also true. "Use it or lose it" isn't just a cute quote; it's a scientific reality where muscles are concerned. You can work your way up to a routine of 5 sets of 20-pound lifts with 10 reps per set, and the minute you switch to 10-pound weights, or 3 sets only, or 8 reps per set, your shock your muscles to adapt downward, and they shrink to the lesser demands placed on them.

So as you go through this chapter and fashion a program to get your shoulders strong and keep them strong for life, it's important to remain mindful of these realities. It's also essential to start slowly, ease back into your exercise program, and keep at it.

THE SUPER-SHOULDER WORKOUTS

This chapter contains three workouts I've devised specifically for people returning to the gym after an injury or shoulder pain—or, of course, in the wake of an illness or other forced absence from exercise. Two of the workouts are at beginner level; both are for easing back into flat-out, intensive muscle work. Why two beginner workouts? Presenting two options is a hedge against boredom, and avoiding boredom is a hedge against neglecting your workout. The fact is that I am going to ask those returning to gym work to stay at this beginner level for at least six months. In preparing two different workouts for those six months, I'm giving you the ability to switch from one to the other. My fear is that when people grow bored with their exercises, they tend to take shortcuts. They try to speed things up, and all too often, they move on to a more advanced level even if they may not be fully ready to do so. In this case, if you get bored with one set of beginner exercises, there's another, and that means there's no excuse for playing fast and loose with the six-month, ease-in period.

But once you've spent half a year doing the beginning workouts, workout number three takes it up a notch.

Beginner or advanced, easing in or steady state, the purpose of these exercise workouts is to grow stronger—specifically, to create what I call super shoulders that can do all the lifting, pushing, pulling, throwing, catching, and hugging you need to do, any way you need to do it—whether up, down, sideways, or across the body—for the rest of your life. Each of the three workouts for ensuring that kind of super shoulder contains a collection of exercises you can choose from. You will be asked to do each a number of times, counted of course as repetitions of the movement.

What everyone always wants to know first is how often to do these exercises and with how much weight. Both are good questions, so let's turn to the answers now.

How Often and With How Much Weight?

Based on both the research I have done and my own experience as a physical therapist working with a varied population, I recommend that you do your super shoulder workout no more than three times a week, leaving at least a full day between workouts. In other words, work out every second day at most. The idea is to give your body a rest in between workouts, and a full day "off" gives the muscles and the surrounding tissue and nerves the rest they need.

Okay, sometimes you miss a workout. You thought you had time to hit the gym this evening, but then your boss asks you to stay late, or a friend calls with a free ticket to that concert you've been dying to go to, or you feel a cold coming on and figure you should get home to bed. Whatever the reason, it's a reminder that we don't really live in a perfect world where nothing ever interferes with our plans.

And then sometimes, you miss the next workout after *that* as well: the cold lingers, the boss again asks you to stay late, there's a movie you're just dying to see.

Now you've missed two workouts in a row, and the tendency is to feel that you've just blown it, it is all too much, and you might as well quit trying to have a regular schedule of workouts. But that kind of thinking is always a mistake.

Please don't quit. Studies have shown that even two workouts a week will give you great results, almost as good as training three times a week.[1] Consistency is really more important than adherence to a perfect schedule. Try for the former, and don't worry if you do not achieve the latter. The results you need and want come from keeping at it, not from being perfect—which no one is, anyway.

On the other side of the coin, let me remind you again of the lesson we learned long ago in this book: the false notion that working harder sooner will make you stronger faster. Unfortunately, the body does not work that way. If you trained every day, your body would never get a chance to rest and grow. Without such rest, you simply become even more vulnerable to injury, and you further postpone the day when you get better and stronger.

To recap: You can build a super shoulder by doing your shoulder workout three times a week with a rest day in between if you can, two times a week with at least one rest day in between if you cannot. But put the emphasis on consistency, not adherence to a schedule.

What Kind of Weights Should You Use at the Beginning?

That is, when you return to the gym and start to ease back into a workout schedule, what kind of weights should you use?

Clearly, there is no single straightforward answer to this. We are all different. Some people are just naturally strong in some areas and naturally weak in others, so for each of us, it's a matter of trial and error. But here is the key: *The aim is to feel the muscle working, not straining.* Too much weight can compromise proper form and technique; too little weight won't constitute a workout.

And just how do you measure what's too much and what's too little? My general rule of thumb is that the "correct" weight is one with which you can comfortably do 8 repetitions but start to strain at more than 10 repetitions. At the very least, when your last rep feels difficult to do, that's probably your limit or one rep over your limit.

Let's say that you are sitting on the bench, ready to perform an exercise called the Seated Bent Over Dumbbell Raise. Holding dumbbells in each hand, you bend forward at the waist, keeping your hands behind your calves. You then lift the weights out to the side as high as you can—slightly higher than the level of your head if possible. Then you slowly lower the weights to your sides.

Simple as it sounds, it's my long-held observation that most people tend to find this exercise tough to do. Perhaps because it is not a movement we naturally do very often, most people are pretty weak in this exercise. So even very fit gym rats who will naturally reach for a 10-pound dumbbell right off the bat, find they can only do half a dozen lifts before their arms start swinging every which way—a clear signal that the weight is in charge, not the muscle. Given our 8-rep standard, that means the 10-pounder is really too heavy.

On the other hand, reaching for a 2-pounder may empower you to do a good 8 reps—even to go beyond 10 reps—but it won't give you a good muscle pump. That means that while you might be increasing your muscle endurance, you won't be doing anything for muscle strength and hypertrophy—that is, for making the muscle grow.

So let's split the difference, more or less. Pick up a 5-pound dumbbell and push out 8 repetitions in good form, then maybe extend two more reps to 10—tough but doable—and that will equate to your ideal starting weight.

Now that you have gotten the exercises from previous chapters, I want to supplement your strength-building program with some great exercises that you can incorporate in the gym. These exercises will definitely help improve your strength and stability and definitely give you the confidence that you need to do things that you didn't think you would ever have the power to do again!

All of these exercises are weight-training exercises, using dumbbells, barbells, or cables. In general, dumbbells give you greater range of motion than a barbell does. They also make you work harder, because unlike the barbell, dumbbells stay straight only because you stabilize them. Another plus, of course, is that it's a bit faster and easier to let a dumbbell drop than a barbell—should it become necessary to do so.

The barbell, on the other hand, offers the advantage that the weight is fixed and stable. There's no deviation, and that makes the barbell easy to work with.

Cable machines enable a kind of flexibility and complexity—the arms can go in different directions at once in a controlled and stable manner, for example—that make it extremely utilitarian, as well as providing a unique "feel" to the kind of resistance you're up against.

So it is useful and indeed desirable to use all three of these technologies in your workouts, if you can. And it's particularly useful to switch from one to the other. Variety is as good for the body as for the psyche. Mixing it up not only keeps you from getting bored with your exercise routine; it's also a great way to challenge the muscles. That's just what these routines try to do.

Some of the exercises in the routines may be new to you, and that's a good thing. Remember: Shock and awe are good for your muscles. Accustomed to training a certain way with a certain weight, they need a jolt to get stronger and tougher.

I offer two pieces of advice for these exercises and for keeping your shoulders strong for life.

First, once you've determined which exercises you find easy and which hard, start your workout with the hard ones first. The beginning of a workout is when your energy level is at its highest. As you probably know, by the end of a workout session, your energy is draining, your mind starts to wander, and you're in danger of losing focus. So it is best to do the tougher exercises up front when they will seem easier to you. In addition, with the easier work at the end, you'll find you can keep going longer.

Second, save the exercises that specifically train the rotator cuff for the end of your workout. I've marked such exercises with an asterisk. These are over and above the primary strengthening of the rotator cuff you did in chapter 4. The point is that you don't want to tire these muscles out at the beginning of your workout and then go on to other exercises that may involve an already fatigued rotator cuff area. That's almost like asking for an injury. Instead, save them for last and take great care to do them with the proper technique, and your rotator cuff will only get stronger and more stable.

Once You've Regained that Strength, Will You Need to Do These Exercises Forever in Order to Prevent Future Injury?

It's a question I am frequently asked, and although no one can predict with certainty what may happen to an individual in the future, the research shows pretty clearly that rotator cuff muscles that start strong require less "repair" from a problem than muscles that have not been exercised. One study back in 2000 demonstrated that once the strength goal for the rotator cuff had been reached, it would need only once-a-week training to keep the gain in strength.[2] There is a catch, however: You have to exercise at the same intensity consistently, every time you are working out the rotator cuff area, so keep that in mind as you perform these exercises and work your way back to full strength.

But the lesson is clear: Exercise is the best way to achieve and maintain a strong set of shoulders for life.

One final but important note: If you are not sure whether or not a particular exercise may be right for you, make sure you ask your doctor or health professional. Only when you are confident that an exercise can help you will you be motivated to do it, and to do it right, and thereby to get stronger. You will feel a whole lot better—and your shoulder will thank you!

BEGINNER EXERCISES

Here are the eight beginner exercises to do as you head back to the gym—
home gyms count too!—to get your shoulder or shoulders back in shape.
Mix and match to create your own program or follow my suggested routine. Either way, stick with these exercises for six months before moving
on to the advanced exercises.

Caution: What is most important with all these exercises is that you
feel the contraction of the muscle you're working. If you don't, stop and
reassess your position. Be sure the weight you are working with is neither
too heavy nor too light. And check your form and technique—in a mirror
if possible or with the help of a fellow-exerciser. If your technique and/or
form are wrong, you're simply cheating the movement and failing to gain
the benefits you seek.

Months 1, 3, 5

*Scaption with a Shrug: 3 × 10
Seated Bent Over Dumbbell Raise: 3 × 10
Standing Cable External Rotation: 3 × 10
Bent Over Cable Lateral: 3 × 10

Months 2, 4, 6

Bent Over Barbell Row: 3 × 10
*Seated One-Arm Cross Cable Lateral: 3 × 10
One-Arm Bent Over Row: 3 × 10
Standing Cable Lateral: 3 × 10
Seated Cable Row: 3 × 10

*Scaption with a Shrug[3]

Scaption is a shortened term for *scapular plane elevation*, which refers
to a particular position in which your arms, with your thumbs up,
are raised out in front of you but at an angle of 30 to 45 degrees,
each arm going toward your side such that your arms end up about
halfway between the front of you and either side of you. When you're

standing thus, you have elevated your arms to the plane of your scapula, and this is your starting position for this exercise.

The Scaption with a Shrug exercise not only increases the size of your shoulders but also powers up your rotator cuff muscles, leading to much stronger shoulder joints. This makes the link to your shoulders a very powerful one, so that your upper body is able to handle greatly increased weight. Here's how to do the exercise:

Grab a pair of dumbbells in a neutral, thumbs-up grip. Start with light weights—maybe three pounds—until you feel comfortable with the movement. Get into position: Stand tall with feet shoulder width apart and arms at your sides with palms facing each other. Raise your arms at a 30- to 45-degree angle until they are at the height of your shoulders at about 90 degrees of flexion in relation to your body. Now shrug your shoulders, trying to raise them up to your ears, while keeping the weights at shoulder height. Return to the starting point to end the repetition.

Your goal: 3 × 10 reps

Watch out for: Don't lift past 90 degrees, and try to keep your wrists straight. Only increase the weight when you are able to do 8 to 10 repetitions smoothly.

Seated Bent Over Dumbbell Raise

This is an exercise that primarily works the back of the shoulder—that is, the posterior deltoid muscle. Sitting on the edge of the bench, dumbbell in each hand, bend forward at the hips, keeping your hands behind your calves. Now, in one second, lift the weights out to the side as high as you can—at least slightly higher than the level of your head. Hold for two seconds, then slowly lower the weight to your sides in a controlled manner over three seconds to finish the repetition.

Your goal: 3 × 10 reps. Remember: one second to lift, two seconds to hold, three seconds to lower.

Watch out for: Too much weight. Proper technique is what counts here, not higher weight levels. Beware also the tendency to cheat on positioning: Keep your arms in line with your shoulders and don't let the weights drift back behind your shoulders. A lift that reaches too far forward will work the front part of your shoulders instead of the back. A lift that goes too far behind you emphasizes your trapezius and your latissimus dorsi muscles, not your rear deltoids, which are the target of the exercise.

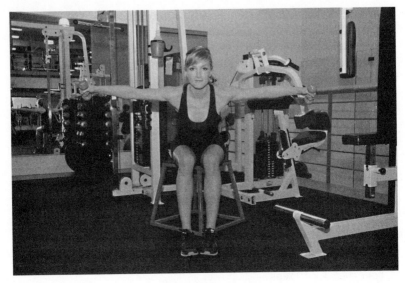

Seated Bent Over Raises

Standing Cable External Rotation

Here is a variation on the exercises from chapter 4 that you did in a
side-lying position with a free weight. Stand sideward to the cable
pulley and a couple of feet away. The cable should be at the height
of your waist. Grasp the cable handle with your opposite or distant
hand, locking your elbow against your side and stretching your
forearm across your waist. Rotate your arm in a backhand motion,
pulling the cable as far as you can across your body while keeping
your elbow tight against your body. Return to the starting position
in a controlled manner.

Be sure to keep your wrist straight at all times, and don't overclench the
handle. The movement should come from the shoulder, not the forearm. You may have to slightly release your elbow as you go through
the movement; otherwise, keep it tight to the body. Stand upright,
eyes straight ahead.

Your goal: 3 × 10 reps

Watch out for: The tendency is to twist the body to help with the movement. Focus on keeping your body as straight as possible facing in
one direction; decrease the weight resistance if necessary to do so.

Bent Over Cable Lateral

This is another cable exercise that will target those rear shoulder muscles. What is unique about this exercise, however, is that you get a bigger range of motion through continuous tension on the muscles involved. You'll use two pulleys from the floor, the right cable in your left hand, the left cable in your right hand. Bend over such that your back is as straight and as parallel to the floor as possible. Then, keeping your arms straight, raise your arms out to either side; do this in one second. The trick is to not extend the arms fully. Instead, keep some tension in them, and hold the position for two seconds. Then take three seconds to slowly return your arms to the starting position.

Your goal: 3 × 10 reps

Watch out for: Your position. Keep your upper body parallel to the floor, and be sure that your knees are slightly bent in order to protect your back.

Bent Over Barbell Row

This is a great exercise for strengthening your rhomboid muscles on both sides—the muscles located between your spine and your shoulder blade, as well as your entire upper back. As an extra added attraction, these Bent Over Barbell Rows also improve your posture, and they're a particularly potent complement to the One-Arm Bent Over Row exercises we'll get to soon. So there's a lot of bang for the buck in this exercise.

Stand with feet shoulder width apart, bend your knees, and with your back as straight as possible, grasp the bar. Your upper body should now be almost parallel to the floor bending at the hips. Think of your arms as hooks, and in one second of time, pull the bar up to your upper abdominals, hold for two seconds, and slowly lower the bar in three seconds. Do not let the bar touch the floor.

Your goal: 3 × 10 reps

Watch out for: Form! Keep your upper back parallel to the floor, hold your spine steady, bend your knees slightly at all times. Also, the lift should extend only as high as your upper abs, not your chest. Lifting up above the abdominals requires you to use your biceps rather than your back and could lead to injury.

*Seated One-Arm Cross Cable Lateral

This exercise will strengthen your rear deltoids, your rotator cuff, and
your rhomboids. It's done seated, facing a floor-level cable pulley.
Grasp the cable handle, make sure your body is stable and still,
then pull the weight up and across your body until the arm is fully
straight out to that side at about shoulder height. Take one second
for the pull, hold for two seconds, and lower to the starting position
in three seconds.

Your goal: 3 ×10 reps

Watch out for: Technique and the amount of weight. Always start with
a lighter weight so that you get the technique right; you'll know it's
right when you feel it in the pertinent areas—deltoids, rotator cuff,
rhomboids. Too much weight can force you to turn your body too
much. This not only makes the exercise useless for its stated pur-
poses, it also could cause injury.

One Arm Bent Over Row

Primarily working your rhomboid muscles, this is a fantastic strengthening exercise that should be part of any exercise routine. There are
varied ways to perform the exercise, but the following is my recom-
mendation.

With a dumbbell in one hand and with the other hand on a bench or
chair for support, bend forward at the hips until the upper part of
your body is almost parallel to the floor. From the starting position—
the weight hanging down—lift the dumbbell up by squeezing your
shoulder blade to your spine, rather than by raising your arm. Take
one second for the lift, hold for two seconds, lower in three seconds.

Your goal: 3 sets × 10 reps on each side

Watch out for: Try not to use your biceps or forearm muscles to do the
work. You want to feel this in the shoulder blade region rather than
in the arm. Make sure you keep the body steady and take care not to
rotate the back when lifting.

Standing Cable Lateral

This is another variation on the Bent Over Cable Lateral, and it is best
performed with one arm at a time. Standing sideways to the cable
machine, grip the handle with the outside hand and pull it across
your body. Keep the tension on your shoulder; don't let the cable
rest against your body.

Your goal: 3 × 10 reps

Watch out for: Make sure that the level of the handle is at the same level as your shoulder. Your working arm should be at approximately 90 degrees to your body when performing that exercise.

Seated Cable Row

This exercise forces the rhomboids to contract at a different angle from their normal contraction, a shock-and-awe move that makes them stronger. Sit at the rowing machine, grip both handles, and, using your rhomboid muscles, pull by squeezing your shoulder blades together as hard as you can. Keep that tension as you "row."

Your goal: 3 × 10 reps

Watch out for: Your elbows and your hands. Hug the elbows to the side of your body and don't let them flare out to the side. And keep your hands in a neutral position while performing the exercise.

ADVANCED EXERCISES

By now, after six months of regular exercising, you have no doubt gained confidence about performing the beginner exercises safely and effectively. At the same time, your shoulder should certainly be back to its base strength. From here on in, the idea is to work toward solidifying that base of strength and building on it. The five exercises of the advanced routine are aimed at doing just that. They constitute one more shock to awe your rotator cuff and shoulder muscles to a peak level of strength and performance. The five advanced exercises are the following:

Front Dumbbell Raise
Dumbbell Presse
Side Lying Lateral Raise
Standing Lateral Raise
*Face Pull

Start with 2 sets of 10 reps each and work your way up to 3 sets.

Front Dumbbell Raise

This exercise strengthens the anterior deltoid head and is very helpful for people who may have partly or completely dislocated a shoulder.

You can do the exercise either seated or standing. I suggest doing it seated because it offers less chance for swinging the weight than the standing position does—and that means less cheating on the movement and on the benefits. Hold a weight in each hand using an overhand grip, hand position at the starting position, and alternate right and left arms as you lift the weight up in a big arc to a point above the top of your head; then bring it slowly down in a controlled manner. The alternating of the pulls means that as you are lifting one dumbbell upward, you are lowering the other.

There are a couple of different ways of doing this exercise. For one thing, rather than an overhand grip, you can use an underhand one—that is, gripping the dumbbells with palms facing downward; this also works the biceps. You can also use a barbell instead of the dumbbells. Hold the bar with palms down and at arm's length resting on your thighs in a standing position. The movement is the same: Lift to a point higher than your head, then lower it all the way in a controlled movement.

Your goal: 2–3 sets × 10 reps

Watch out for: To get the full benefit of this exercise, make sure the weight passes in front of your face rather than beside your body on both the lift and the lowering. That positioning produces a much better contraction in the deltoid.

Dumbbell Press

Pressing weight up over your head, typically using a barbell, is the classic weight-training exercise—the so-called Military Press. But it can actually be a dangerous exercise because of the tendency to bring the bar behind the neck, which in turn means arching the back, all of which can be harmful. So I prefer using dumbbells to do presses.

Seated, hold the dumbbells at shoulder height with your arms open to the side at 90 degrees to your body, elbows out to the sides and palms facing forward. Keeping your back straight, lift the dumbbells up and toward each other until they touch or almost touch at the top of the movement. Lower in a controlled manner. It is not unlikely that you will find it harder to lower the dumbbells than to lift them, but it is very important to do this eccentric phase of the repetition slowly and deliberately. Most people don't. They almost drop the dumbbells, letting them go with a jerk to the body. Little wonder many people develop strains and other injuries in doing this exercise—the consequences of doing it incorrectly.

Your goal: 2–3 sets × 10 reps

Watch out for: Arching your back, especially as you start to increase the amount of weight you lift. A slight, momentary arching movement may be needed to help you push the weight up past the sticking point, but too much arching will in time develop into back pain, and no one wants that.

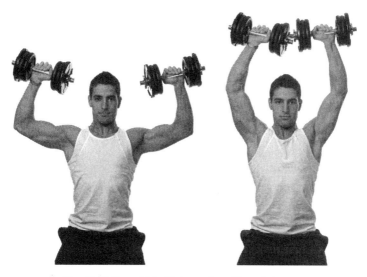

Dumbbell Press. *Nickp37, image from Bigstockphoto.com*

Side Lying Lateral Raise

This is a great way to strengthen the rear and side deltoids. Keep the weights on the light side (about 3–5 pounds) for this movement, and follow the instructions for each step of the movement with strict discipline; no cheating.

Lie on your side on an abdominal board or an incline bench at an angle of 45 degrees to the floor. Your feet are more or less touching the floor. Keeping the head supported is essential; if you don't, your neck will bother you eventually. Grasp the dumbbell in the uppermost hand, bend your elbow slightly, and lower the weight all the way to the floor, making sure you don't twist your wrist inward. Then quickly raise the weight as high up as you can, and slowly lower it back to the floor.

Your goal: 2–3 sets × 10 reps each arm

Watch out for: Your wrists. Keep them straight. Although it has been shown that turning your hand inward as if you are pouring a glass of water will effect a tighter contraction of the muscle, it can also create an impingement problem—and accompanying pain—precisely what you are trying to avoid.

Standing Lateral Raise

Hold a dumbbell in each hand to the side of your body, then bring the weights together in front of your body with palms facing each other. Lean forward a bit, and with a slight bend in your elbow, lift your arms to your side at an angle of 90 degrees or to shoulder height. Now lower your arms slowly, resisting gravity just a little bit all the way down.

Your goal: 2–3 sets × 10 reps

Look out for: Your wrists and gravity. As with the Side Lying Raises, it's all too easy to turn your hands over as if pouring water out of a glass, but you have had a shoulder injury or shoulder pain, and that argues against that movement. Its excessive internal rotation can lead to pinching and impingement, and that's something you don't want to go back to. Beware also the tendency to let momentum move the weights; make sure you're not rocking the weight back and forth and swinging the dumbbell upward. Your deltoids have to do the work. Make them lift the dumbbells themselves. Try a smaller weight if this is a problem. Remember that the exercise is about feeling the muscle working, not about how many pounds you are lifting.

Face Pull*

This is probably the most underrated exercise in strength training. In fact, I'll lay odds that most people haven't even heard of the Face Pull. Yet it is a movement that not only strengthens your back and shoulder—especially the rotator cuff muscles—but also develops balance throughout the region. Specifically, the Face Pull develops the middle and lower trapezius muscles; it strengthens the external rotators of the shoulder; it works the upper rotators of the shoulder, and this counterbalances the dominant downward rotators. The result is a much better and more stable balance in the shoulder.

The Face Pull is called that because your face is the "destination" of the pull, sort of. Here's how to do it: You're going to be pulling at a two-handled rope or cable, so the first thing to do is to adjust the handle on the machine to be at your eye level. Stand a few feet away. Using a neutral grip—that is, with your thumbs pointed up—pull the rope or cable all the way to your ears, past your face. Your arms are now perpendicular to your body, elbows out, while the neutral grip ensures that you have performed an external rotation movement to strengthen and stabilize the shoulder.

Your goal: 2–3 sets × 10 reps

Watch out for: The position of your pecs. In order to get the most out of this exercise, make sure you stick your chest out throughout the movement. Think of the movement not as a pull on the cable handles but rather as squeezing your shoulder blades together. That's where you really get the benefit of this essential exercise.

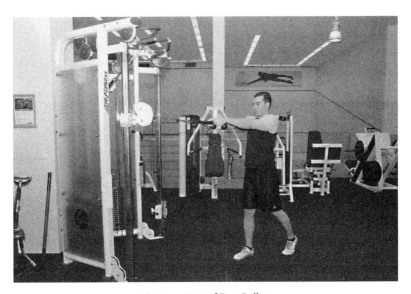

Start position of Face Pulls

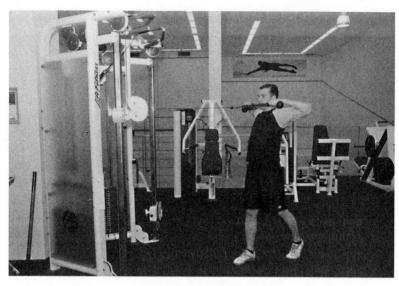

End position of Face Pulls

There might be some more variations of these exercises that you can do for your rotator cuff. As long as you perform them with the proper technique, you will only get stronger and your rotator cuff will become more stable. If you are not sure if an exercise is right for you, make sure you ask your doctor or your allied health professional. Knowing that the proper exercise will help you will be a great motivator to your getting better as quickly as possible. You will feel a whole lot better and your shoulder will really thank you.

TRAINING YOUR SHOULDER FOR SPECIFIC SPORTS

We all have our favorite sport. It helps us unwind, release stress, and lets us have some fun again. But suffering from a rotator cuff or shoulder problem might stop us from participating in something that we truly love.

If you are still suffering from your tendonitis or other shoulder problem, please refer to chapter 4 to find exercises to build your strength and range of motion to acceptable levels. Below are some of the exercises done for general conditioning in the gym, but now applied specifically to your favorite sport. These exercise programs are just a small sample of the many different exercises one can do. While most of these exercises are done with free weights, you can use elastic bands, kettle balls, or any other type of weight to get the effect that you are looking for.

Note: These are advanced routines. I do not suggest performing them until you can safely do the exercise routines listed in chapter 4, as well as the gym routines listed previously in this chapter. You should only proceed with the exercises and routines listed below when you are confident with your performance of the exercise routines in this chapter.

Baseball/Softball

It is well known that constantly throwing a baseball, as a pitcher does, can develop shoulder problems. Shoulder impingement pain and rotator cuff injuries are probably the most commonly seen injuries in baseball, softball, or any throwing sport, regardless of the player's age or level of play.

Pitchers in baseball have worse rotator cuff problems than softball players due to the way the ball is thrown. The difference is due to the overhead throwing motion versus the underhand throwing motion. Do you know why pitchers in baseball have their pitches counted? It is due to the potential of a rotator cuff injury if too many pitches are thrown.

The motion of throwing a ball has five stages. I would like to focus on the deceleration part of a throw or slowing the throwing arm down. When you decelerate the arm, your elbow extends while your shoulder, specifically your rotator cuff, contracts to try to absorb the violent forces placed on it—especially if you want to impress your team with your killer fastball. Problems will begin to arise if your rotator cuff muscles and supporting muscles are not strong enough. By properly strengthening your shoulder muscles, creating a balance among the front, side, and back parts of your shoulder (as well as the rest of your body), you can impress the people around you with your blazing powerful throws, while also avoiding the much-dreaded disabled list.

Baseball/Softball Exercises

1. Across the Body Stretch: 2 × 1 minute
2. Doorway Chest Stretch: 2 × 1 minute
3. Bent Over Dumbbell Flys: 3 × 10
4. Superman: 2 × 10

5. Front Raise: 2 × 10
6. Scaption with a Shrug: 2 × 10
7. Face Pull: 2 × 10
8. Standing Cable External Rotation: 2 × 10

Golf

Do golfers really get injured? Although golf may look like a gentle, low-risk sport, studies have shown that amateur and professional golfers on average suffer two injuries per year. If you swing the golf club using an improper technique (I might have experienced that) you can definitely get an overuse injury. Even though shoulder issues are not the highest with pro tour golfers, a vast majority of players suffer rotator cuff impingement injuries. Studies have shown that it is the lead shoulder that is often involved with a large range of motion during the swing and is often injured. If your rotator cuff muscles are not strengthened they will have to contract harder than they should just to stabilize your humeral head in the glenohumeral (G/H) joint. Atrophy of your rotator cuff muscles can occur in older golfers. Due to the repetition of the golf swing, imbalanced or weak stabilizing shoulder muscles can cause impingement, degeneration, or even rotator cuff tears. Therefore balancing the shoulder muscles, from front to back, should be the main focus of a rotator cuff program.

Golf Exercises

1. Doorway Chest Stretch: 2 × 1 min.
2. Thoracic Extension Mobilization Exercise: 1 × 10 with 5 second hold
3. Airplane: 2 × 10
4. Superman: 2 × 10
5. Sitting Abduction with Alphabet: 1 × 1 alphabet
6. Seated One-Arm Cross Cable Lateral: 2 × 10
7. Bent Over Barbell Row: 2 × 10
8. Dumbbell Press: 2 × 10

Tennis

Tennis is an amazing sport. I have worked in two Olympics just to have the amazing opportunity to treat some of the finest tennis players in the world. I can tell you from personal experience that 80–90 percent of the players participating in these tournaments are playing with some kind of injury. Shoulder injuries are very common to tennis players, as repetitive motions such as the serve can cause an overuse injury if you are not careful. Again, a weak rotator cuff might be the culprit. Your backhand might place your shoulder joint at awkward angles.

Remember how hard you hit the ball when you serve at high speeds and at the extreme ranges of motion. It has been said that the overhead motion of a tennis serve might almost look like the same movement as throwing a fastball in baseball. When you serve, your rib cage tilts to the side, your shoulder blade starts to go outward or abduct, and your arm and shoulder might go to more than 100 degrees of external rotation. Wow! If you do not strengthen your back muscles, including your rhomboids, traps, and serratus anterior, as well as your rotator cuff, injuries to your shoulder can happen. Here is a good sample exercise routine that can really help your tennis game.

Tennis Exercises

1. Doorway Chest Stretch: 2 × 1 min.
2. Across the Body Stretch: 2 × 1 min.
3. Shoulder Blade Push-Up: 2 × 10
4. Side Lying External Rotation: 2 × 10
5. Side Lying Alphabet: 1 × 1 alphabet
6. Bent Over Barbell Row: 2 × 10
7. Standing Cable External Rotation: 2 × 10
8. Seated One-Arm Cross Cable Lateral: 2 × 10

Football

American football, not to be confused with international football or what is called *soccer* in North America, is a great sport. The attention that the Super Bowl gets, the National Football League's (NFL) championship game is astounding. Shoulder injuries are very common in football, ranging from acromioclavicular (A/C) sprains to shoulder dislocations, anterior and posterior. Studies show that an acute shoulder dislocation is really an anterior dislocation of the glenohumeral joint of the shoulder. This happens when a runner or tackler gets his arm in a forced outstretched position with a forced external rotation. Seen primarily in offensive linemen, a posterior dislocation can also happen when the shoulder blade is pushed backward and, with repetitive trauma, the shoulder partially dislocates, or subluxates, or completely dislocates. As with all the other exercises that we have spoken about, strengthening your shoulder muscles—from the rotator cuff to the deltoid and supporting muscles—is a must. Here is a sample routine that can build strength quickly and safely.

Football Exercises

1. Face Pull: 2 × 10
2. Bent Over Barbell Row: 2 × 20
3. Side Lying Alphabet with 5 lbs.: 2 × 10
4. Standing Cable External Rotation: 2 × 10
5. Dumbbell Press: 2 × 10
6. Lateral Raise: 2 × 10
7. Front Raise: 2 × 10
8. Bent Over Rear Flys: 2 × 10

Swimming

I find that swimming injuries are a little different from the other sports I mentioned because they are more chronic than acute in nature, but they still result from repetitive movements with overused muscles. Shoulder problems in swimmers are caused by repeating the same movements, sometimes incorrect mechanics that cause fatigue, and strain on the rotator cuff muscles as well as the long head of the biceps. These problems normally happen in the butterfly or freestyle/crawl swimming, when the arm is in forward, flexed, abducted, and internally rotated position. They can also happen in the backstroke, because the arms provide 75 percent propulsion in the stroke. If your muscles in the opposite direction, especially your external rotators, cannot counterbalance this movement, then a cuff or even bicep impingement might happen.

A rotator cuff injury in a swimmer sometimes referred to as *swimmer's shoulder* is found in about 60 percent of professional competitive swimmers. I think that it should be called a *swimmer's friction shoulder* due to all the rubbing that the rotator cuff muscles and biceps tendon get from repeated stroke movement. A backstroke swimmer can also possibly get some instability in the front of their shoulder due to all the backward arm movement while they swim. The most common time to feel pain is during the pull phase of the stroke. You might feel or hear clicking in the shoulder, which tells that an injury is developing.

A strong rotator cuff can significantly reduce the discomfort in your shoulder. But you should also work your rhomboids, trapezius, and serratus anterior muscles, located on and around the shoulder blade to ensure optimal efficient movement and decrease injuries. Stretching before swimming can also help, with warming up your muscle-tendon units so they do not feel tight when they are about to go in the water. Just be careful that you don't overstretch the anterior part of your shoulder.

If you feel deep pain, don't let it go, please see your doctor or your physical therapist. If these types of injuries are left untreated, they can lead to rotator cuff tears.

Studies have shown that strokes that are done with a recovery underwater, such as a breaststroke are actually easier on the shoulder. I personally prefer that you do breaststroke rather than the crawl stroke. It is to your benefit to work on your technique and your kicks as opposed to high-volume type of swimming. Here is a sample exercise swimming program:

Swimming Exercises

1. Across the Body Stretch: 2 × 1 min.
2. Side Lying External Rotation: 2 × 10
3. Side Lying Lifting Arm Straight Up: 2 × 10
4. Side Lying Alphabet: 1 × 1 alphabet
5. Bent Over Barbell Row: 2 × 10
6. Shoulder Blade Push-Up: 2 × 10
7. Scaption with a Shrug: 2 × 10
8. Face Pull: 2 × 10

Basketball

Although it is commonly known that knee and ankle injuries take center stage when a person plays basketball, rotator cuff injuries present themselves frequently as well. These are common from doing too many repetitive movements like shooting and shot blocking. Over time, imbalances in your shoulder will start to creep up on you, causing you pain and making you want to stop playing for a while. Strengthening your shoulder is the best way to decrease and possibly eliminate shoulder tendinitis. Here is a sample basketball program:

Basketball Exercises

1. Doorway chest stretch: 2 × 1 min.
2. Side Lying External Rotation: 2 × 10
3. Side Lying Lifting Arm Straight Up: 2 × 10
4. Sitting Abduction with Alphabet: 2 × 1 alphabet
5. Standing Cable External Rotations: 2 × 10
6. Seated One-Arm Cross Cable Laterals: 2 × 10
7. Superman: 2 × 10
8. Bent Over Cable Flys: 2 × 10

Hockey

Hockey is considered Canada's national sport but it is played in countries all over the world. Shoulder injuries from hockey tend to be more traumatic in nature, normally in the form of some kind of dislocation. The most common type of separation is the A/C separation, where the ligament holding the acromion to the clavicle is stretched, pulled, or torn. This is the same as stating that you might have a grade 1, 2 or 3 A/C separation. If you have a grade 3 separation, you would need surgery to fix that, but let the doctor and medical team advise you on that. Studies have shown that 45 percent of all hockey players have experienced some level of arthritis in that area. A good shoulder routine is an excellent way to decrease any chance of injury to your shoulder.

Hockey Exercises

1. Across the body stretch: 2 × 1 min.
2. Airplane: 2 × 10
3. Face Pull: 2 × 10
4. Sitting Flexion: 2 × 10
5. Scaption with a Shrug: 2 × 10
6. Bent Over Barbell Row: 2 × 10
7. Dumbbell Press: 2 × 10
8. Standing Cable External Rotation: 2 × 10

Gymnastics

A very popular sport for men as well as women, gymnatics requires lots of different components to do well in these events. It is interesting to note that different shoulder injuries will happen on the most part, to men than women. Habitual repetitive training causes tightening of the internal rotators of the shoulder—mainly the pecs, lats, anterior deltoid, teres major, and long head of the biceps muscle for women. It has been shown that many female gymnasts have poor shoulder flexibility and almost no external rotation, which can lead to bad rotator cuff issues. While men can have the same issues as women, men performing the rings actually opens up the shoulders a little too much, creating too much range of motion and not enough stability. A balanced shoulder program for both men and women can really help them excel in their sport.

Gymnastic Exercises for Women

1. Across the Body Stretch: 2 × 1 min.
2. Thoracic Extension Mobilization Exercise: 1 × 10 × 5 sec hold
3. Doorway Chest Stretch: 2 × 1 min.
4. Standing Cable External Rotations: 2 × 10
5. Side Lying Lifting Arm Straight Up: 2 × 10
6. Side Lying Alphabet: 1 × 1 alphabet
7. Face Pulls: 2 × 10
8. Bent Over Rows: 2 × 10

Gymnastic Exercises for Men

1. Side Lying External Rotation: 2 × 10
2. Side Lying Lifting Arm Straight Up: 2 × 10
3. Side Lying Alphabet: 1 × 1 alphabet
4. One-Arm Bent Over Row: 2 × 10 each side
5. Face Pulls: 2 × 10
6. Rear Delt Flys: 2 × 10
7. Side Lying Lateral Raises: 2 × 10
8. Scaption with a Shrug: 2 × 10

Construction Job

Construction workers use their shoulders a lot to do their job and shoulder injuries are one of the most common injuries that workers suffer from. Injuries can either be traumatic (for example, resulting from a fall) or due to improper repetitive movements done on a daily basis. People who are particularly prone to injuries include those who have to do work above their heads—that is, painting, drywall installation, plastering, sheet metal work and more. One way to avoid these problems is to really take special care and balance out the shoulders with exercises.

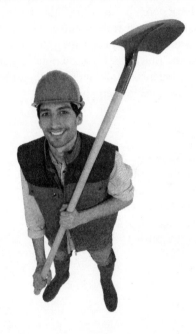

Construction worker.
Auremar, image from Bigstockphoto.com

Construction Job Exercises

1. Standing Cable External Rotation: 2 × 10
2. Face Pull: 2 × 10
3. Dumbbell Press: 2 × 10
4. Shoulder Blade Push-Up: 2 × 10
5. Bent Arm One-Arm Row: 2 × 10
6. Chest Doorway Stretch: 2 × 1 min.
7. Scaption with a Shrug: 2 × 10
8. Seated One-Arm Cross Cable Lateral: 2 × 10

Desk Job

The granddaddy of them all. Sitting at your desk all day using your mouse shouldn't give you problems. You are just sitting quietly doing your job or homework on your computer or at your desk. The problem, as we have discussed in earlier chapters is your posture, as well as your arch-enemy, gravity. When your head is too far forward and your arm is straight in front of you, it is only a matter of time until you start to develop shoulder, neck, and back pain. Making yourself aware of good posture while at your desk is only half the battle. A balanced program should take care of shoulder issues and allow you to work properly.

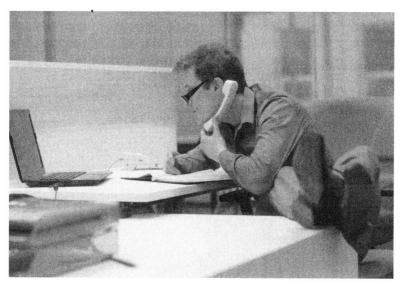

Overworked man at a desk job. *Endomotion, image from Bigstockphoto.com*

Desk Job Exercises

1. Across the Body Stretch: 2 × 1 min.
2. Thoracic Extension Mobilization Exercise: 1 × 10 × 5 sec hold
3. Side Lying External Rotation: 2 × 10
4. Side Lying Lifting Arm Straight Up: 2 × 10
5. Side Lying Alphabet: 1 × 1 alphabet
6. Scaption with a Shrug: 2 × 10
7. Bent Over Rows: 2 × 10
8. Face Pull: 2 × 10

As you can see, your fate does not have to include living with a bad shoulder with nothing else that can be done. By really understanding what is causing your pain and the reasons behind it, you can empower yourself into helping yourself. By having a healthy diet and exercising on a regular basis, as well as quickly addressing problems with the aid of your doctor and your allied health professional before those problems get worse, you can definitely help improve the quality of your shoulders and start enjoying life to the fullest.

Notes

CHAPTER ONE

1. Bahram Jam, "The Shoulder Complex" (Thornhil, ON: Advance Physical Therapy Education Institute, 2000).

2. In fact, the position of the rib cage can be related to shoulder pain. Because it is connected to the thoracic spine, the rib cage has less mobility than the neck or lower back, but it is very strong and stable. As we also noted, the rib cage and the scapula make up the scapulothoracic or S/T joint. For the S/T joint to move properly and efficiently, the rib cage that the scapula slides along must be in its ideal position. If not, that will affect the position of the scapula, which may then slide in an off-kilter way and impinge the shoulder. A research study found that patients with shoulder problems exhibit less thoracic spine mobility in extension (bending backward rather than forward) compared to people with no shoulder problems. Greater mobility in extension in the thoracic spine helps not only breathing but also shoulder and neck problems.

3. G. David et al., "EMG and Strength Correlates of Selected Shoulder Muscles during Rotations of the Glenohumeral Joint," *Clinical Biomechanics* 15, no. 2 (2000): 95–102.

4. Jam, APTEI Course: The Shoulder Complex, lecture notes.

5. G. David et al., "EMG and Strength Correlates," 95–102.

6. P. Ludewig and T. Cook, "Alterations in Shoulder Kinematics and Associated Muscle Activity in People with Symptoms of Shoulder Impingement," *Physical Therapy* 80, no. 3 (2000): 277–91.

CHAPTER TWO

1. J. Scott McMonagle and Emily N. Vinson, "MRI of the Shoulder: Rotator Cuff," *Applied Radiology* 41, no. 4 (2012): 20–27.

2. Surgery may prove a more cost-effective treatment for repair of a full thickness tear than nonsurgical approaches, according to the most recent thinking. Surgery, especially for younger patients, may cost less in the end, "taking into account the indirect costs incurred over a patient's lifetime," although it also cautions that all cases should be considered individually, *The Journal of Bone and Joint Surgery*, 2013.

3. Shoulder impingement syndrome or subacromial syndrome was first described by Dr. Charles Neer in 1972. Asserting that the shape of the acromion, particularly the anterior third section, caused 95 percent of rotator cuff problems, Neer advocates for surgery as the best alternative to relieve the problem. There are actually four types of acromion process. The three classic types, described by Bigliani et al. in "The Morphology of the Acromion and Its Relationship to Rotator Cuff Tears," *Orthopaedic Transactions* 10, no. 228 (1986): 216, are: stage 1) flat, stage 2) curved, and stage 3) hooked. A stage 4 is convex, according to O. Cagey et al. in "Anatomic Basis of Ligamentous Control of Elevation of the Shoulder (Reference Position of the Shoulder Joint)," *Surgical Radiology Anatomy* 9, no. 1 (1987): 19–26. If the shape of the acromion is responsible for impingement problems, then the surgical intervention should be positive for patients, and this has not been the case.

4. A study by J. P. Haahr et al., "Exercises Versus Arthroscopic Decompression in Patients with Subacromial Impingement: A Randomized, Controlled Study in 90 Cases with a One Year Follow Up," *Annals of the Rheumatic Diseases* 64, no. 5 (2005): 760–64, compares physiotherapy and arthroscopic surgical decompression of 90 patients with the sourcil sign (SIS)/rotator cuff pathology. The sourcil sign, seen in an X-ray, is considered an indicator of rotator cuff pathology due to the increased pressure under the acromion, according to Chris Smith et al., "The Sourcil Sign: A Useful Finding on Plain X-ray," *Shoulder & Elbow* 2, no. 1 (2010): 9.

Physiotherapy used pain-relief techniques plus scapular and rotator cuff exercises, whereas the arthroscopic surgical decompression used bursectomy, acromioplasty, partial removal of the coracoacromial ligament, and a physiotherapy program. After a twelve-month follow-up of patients, there was improvement in both groups, no real significant differences for any variables of interest, and some deterioration in a number of patients in both groups. Based on these outcomes, some doctors are reluctant to operate on patients with a Neer stage 2 impingement syndrome.

A study by J. Brox et al., "Arthroscopic Surgery Versus Supervised Exercises in Patients with Rotator Cuff Disease (Stage II Impingement Syndrome): A Prospective, Randomized Controlled Study in 125 Patients with a 2½ Year Follow-Up," *Journal of Shoulder and Elbow Surgery* 8, no. 2 (1999): 102–11 shows that patients with a stage 2 impingement syndrome improved with exercises alone, while surgical treatment to a rotator cuff impingement syndrome shows no better outcomes than physiotherapy with training, according to J. P. Haahr et al., "Exercises Versus Arthroscopic Decompression," 760–64.

CHAPTER THREE

1. J. C. Segen, *The Dictionary of Modern Medicine* (Dictionary Series) (New York: CRC Press, 1992).

2. C. Speed and B. L. Hazelman, "Shoulder Pain," Online version of BMJ's *Clinical Evidence* 2006, accessed February 2006.

3. Amy Myszko, "Vitamins and Minerals that Aid in Collagen Formation," article updated February 5, 2014, accessed May 28, 2014, http://www.livestrong.com/article/357927-supplements-that-re-buildcollagen/.

4. Nanna Goldman et al., "Adenosine A1 Receptors Mediate Local Anti-Nociceptive Effects of Acupuncture," *Nature Neuroscience* 13, no. 7 (2010): 883–88, doi: 10.1038/nn.2562.

5. Joseph H. Pilates, "Bodily House-Cleaning through Circulation," in *Return to Life through Contrology*, (1945; repr., Miami, FL: Pilates Method Alliance, 2005), 27.

6. Pilates, "Bodily House-Cleaning through Circulation," 24.

7. Pilates, "Bodily House-Cleaning through Circulation," 27.

8. Pilates, "Bodily House-Cleaning through Circulation," 24.

CHAPTER FOUR

1. W. Bandy and J. Irion, "The Effect of Time on Static Stretch on the Flexibility of the Hamstring Muscles," *Physical Therapy* 74, no. 9 (1994): 845–52.

2. G. Grimby et al., "Muscle Strength and Endurance after Training with Repeated Maximal Isometric Contraction," *Scandanavian Journal of Rehabilitation Medicine* 5, no. 3 (1973): 118–23.

CHAPTER FIVE

1. I. Kapandji, *The Physiology of the Joints*, Vol. 3 (London: Churchill Livingstone, 1970).

2. R. Caillet and L. Gross, *The Rejuvenation Strategy* (New York: Doubleday and Company, 1987).

3. Dana R. Carney, Amy J. C. Cuddy, and Andy J. Yap, "Power Posing: Brief Nonverbal Displays Affect Neuroendocrine Levels and Risk Tolerance," *Psychological Science* 21, no. 10 (2010).

4. F. Kendall, E. McCreary, and P. Provance, *Muscles, Testing and Function*, 4th ed. (Philadelphia, PA: Lippincott Williams & Wilkins, 1993).

5. J. Marquardt, "Carpal Tunnel Targets Left-handed People," All Stop: Carpal Tunnel Articles, http://allstop.com/carpal-tunnel-articles/carpal-tunnel-and-left-handed-people.html.

CHAPTER SEVEN

1. P. DeMichele et al., "Isometric Torso Rotation Strength: Effect of Training Frequency on Its Development," *Archive Physical Medical Rehabilitation* 78, no. 1 (1997): 64–69; and T. Carroll et al., "Resistance Training Frequency: Strength and Myosin Heavy Chain Responses to Two and Three Bouts per Week," *European Journal of Applied Physiology and Occupational Physiology* 78, no. 3 (1998): 270–75.

2. M. J. McCarrick and J. G. Kemp, "The Effect of Strength Training and Reduced Training on Rotator Cuff Musculature," *Clinical Biomechanics* 15, suppl. 1 (2000): S42–S45.

3. Remember, an asterisk indicates that an exercise specifically trains the rotator cuff.

Bibliography

CHAPTER ONE

David, G., M. E. Magarey, M. A. Jones, Z. Dvir, K. S. Türker, and M. Sharpe. "EMG and Strength Correlates of Selected Shoulder Muscles during Rotations of the Glenohumeral Joint." *Clinical Biomechanics* 15, no. 2 (2000): 95–102.

Jam, Bahram. "The Shoulder Complex." Thornhil, ON: Advance Physical Therapy Education Institute, 2000.

Ludewig, P., and T. Cook. "Alterations in Shoulder Kinematics and Associated Muscle Activity in People with Symptoms of Shoulder Impingement." *Physical Therapy* 80, no. 3 (2000): 277–91.

CHAPTER TWO

Bigliani, L. U., D. Morrison, and E. W. April. "The Morphology of the Acromion and Its Relationship to Rotator Cuff Tears." *Orthopaedic Transactions* 10, no. 228 (1986).

Brox, J., E. Gjengedal, G. Uppheim, A. S. Bøhmer, J. I. Brevik, A. E. Ljunggren, and P. H. Staff. "Arthroscopic Surgery Versus Supervised Exercises in Patients with Rotator Cuff Disease (Stage II Impingement Syndrome): A Prospective, Randomized Controlled Study in 125 Patients with a 2½ Year Follow-Up." *Journal of Shoulder and Elbow Surgery* 8, no. 2 (1999): 102–11.

Cagey, O., H. Bonfait, C. Cillot, I. Hureau, and F. Mazas. "Anatomic Basis of Ligamentous Control of Elevation of the Shoulder (Reference Position of the Shoulder Joint)." *Surgical Radiology Anatomy* 9, no. 1 (1987): 19–26.

Haahr, J. P., S. Østergaard, J. Dalsgaard, K. Norup, P. Frost, S. Lausen, E. A. Holm, and J. H. Andersen. "Exercises Versus Arthroscopic Decompression in Patients with Subacromial Impingement: A Randomized, Controlled Study in 90 Cases with a One Year Follow Up." *Annals of the Rheumatic Diseases* 64, no. 5 (2005): 760–64.

McMonagle, J. Scott, and Emily N. Vinson. "MRI of the Shoulder: Rotator Cuff." *Applied Radiology* 41, no. 4 (2012): 20–27.

Smith, Chris, Rupen Dattani, Victoria Deans, and Steve Drew. "The Sourcil Sign: A Useful Finding on Plain X-ray." *Shoulder & Elbow* 2, no. 1 (2010): 9–12.

CHAPTER THREE

Freidman, Philip, and Gail Eisen, *The Pilates Method of Physical and Mental Conditioning.* New York: Viking Studio, 2005.

Goldman, Nanna, Michael Chen, Takumi Fujita, Qiwu Xu, Weiguo Peng, Wei Liu, Tina K Jensen, Yong Pei, Fushun Wang, Xiaoning Han, Jiang-Fan Chen, Jurgen Schnermann, Takahiro Takano, Lane Bekar, Kim Tieu, and Maiken Nedergaard. "Adenosine A1 Receptors Mediate Local Anti-Nociceptive Effects of Acupuncture." *Nature Neuroscience* 13, no. 7 (2010): 883–88. doi: 10.1038/nn.2562.

Myszko, Amy. "Vitamins and Minerals that Aid in Collagen Formation." Article updated February 5, 2014. Accessed May 28, 2014. http://www.livestrong.com/article/357927–supplements-that-re-buildcollagen/.

Molsberger, A. F., T. Schneider, H. Gotthardt, and A. Drabik. "German Randomized Acupuncture Trial for Chronic Shoulder Pain (GRASP)—A Pragmatic, Controlled, Patient-Blinded, Multi-Centre Trial in an Outpatient Care Environment." *Pain* 151, no. 1 (2010): 146–51.

Pilates, Joseph H. *Return to Life through Contrology.* 1945. Reprint, Miami, FL: Pilates Method Alliance, 2005.

Segen, J. C. *The Dictionary of Modern Medicine* (Dictionary Series). New York: CRC Press, 1992.

Speed, C., and B. L. Hazelman. "Shoulder Pain." Online version of BMJ's *Clinical Evidence* (2006). Accessed February 2006.

CHAPTER FOUR

Bandy, W., and J. Irion. "The Effect of Time on Static Stretch on the Flexibility of the Hamstring Muscles." *Physical Therapy* 74, no. 9 (1994): 845–52.

Garfinkel, S., and E. Carafelli. "Relative Changes in Maximal Force, EMG, and Muscle Cross-Sectional Area after Isometric Training." *Medicine and Science in Sports and Exercise* 24, no. 11 (1992): 1220–27.

Grimby, G., C. Heijne, O. Hook, and H. Wedel. "Muscle Strength and Endurance after Training with Repeated Maximal Isometric Contraction." *Scandanavian Journal of Rehabilitation Medicine* 5, no. 3 (1973): 118–23.

CHAPTER FIVE

Caillet, R., and L. Gross. *The Rejuvenation Strategy.* New York: Doubleday and Company, 1987.

Carney, Dana R., Amy J. C. Cuddy, and Andy J. Yap. "Power Posing: Brief Nonverbal Displays Affect Neuroendocrine Levels and Risk Tolerance." *Psychological Science* 21, no. 10 (2010): 1363–68.

Kapandji, I. *The Physiology of the Joints.* Vol. 3. London: Churchill Livingstone, 1970.

Kendall, F., E. McCreary, and P. Provance. *Muscles, Testing and Function.* 4th ed. Philadelphia, PA: Lippincott Williams & Wilkins, 1993.

Marquardt, J. "Carpal Tunnel Targets Left-handed People." All Stop: Carpal Tunnel Articles. http://allstop.com/carpal-tunnel-articles/carpal-tunnel-and-left-handed-people.html.

CHAPTER SEVEN

Carroll, T. J., P. J. Abernethy, P. A. Logan, M. Barber, and M. T. McEniery. "Resistance Training Frequency: Strength and Myosin Heavy Chain Responses to Two and Three Bouts per Week." *European Journal of Applied Physiology and Occupational Physiology* 78, no. 3 (1998): 270–75.

DeMichele, P. L., M. L. Pollock, J. E. Graves, D. N. Foster, D. Carpenter, L. Garzarella, W. Brechue, and M. Fulton. "Isometric Torso Rotation Strength: Effect of Training Frequency on Its Development." *Archive Physical Medical Rehabilitation* 78, no. 1 (1997): 64–69.

McCarrick, M. J., and J. G. Kemp. "The Effect of Strength Training and Reduced Training on Rotator Cuff Musculature." *Clinical Biomechanics* 15, suppl. 1 (2000): S42–S45.

Index

AAOS. *See* American Academy of Orthopaedic Surgeons
abdominal crunches, 105
abduction, 2, 3
acromioclavicular (A/C) joint, 3, 4, 113
acromion, 152n3
acromion process, 2, 152n3
acupuncture, 52–53
acute injury, 47
acute tear, 20
adduction, 3; horizontal, 68
adhesive capsulitis (frozen shoulder), xiv, 14–16, 35
advanced exercises: Dumbbell Press, 135, 136–37, *137*; Face Pull, 135, 138–39, *139, 140*; Front Dumbbell Raise, 135–36; overview, 135, 140; Side Lying Lateral Raise, 135, 137–38; Standing Lateral Raise, 135, 138. *See also* sports exercises
age, 18
Airplane Exercise, 78–79, *79*
Alphabet with Your Arm at Side in Sitting, 82–83
American Academy of Orthopaedic Surgeons (AAOS), 19

anteriorly tipped pelvis, 102
Arm Across Chest Stretch, 68–69, *69*
Arm to Your Side in Sitting, 82
arthrograms, 35
arthroscopic surgical decompression, 152n4
articular side tears, 19–20

barbells, 128; Barbell Behind-The-Neck Press, 116–17; Bent Over Barbell Row, 130, 133
baseball exercises, 141–42
basketball exercises, 145–46
beginner exercises: Bent Over Barbell Row, 130, 133; Bent Over Cable Lateral, 130, 133; One Arm Bent Over Row, 130, 134; overview, 130; Scaption with a Shrug, 130–31; Seated Bent Over Dumbbell Raise, 130, 131, *132*; Seated Cable Row, 130, 135; Seated One-Arm Cross Cable Lateral, 130, 134; Standing Cable External Rotation, 130, 132; Standing Cable Lateral, 130, 134–35
Bench Press: Dumbbell, 119; Neck, 119–20

bent over exercises: Bent Over Arm Swings and Circles, 66–67; Bent Over Barbell Row, 130, 133; Bent Over Cable Lateral, 130, 133; Seated Bent Over Dumbbell Raise, 130, 131, *132*

biceps, 8–9

biomechanical injuries, 18

bones, 2

bra, posture, 109

brachial plexus, 119

breathing, 23–24

bursa, 12

bursal type tears, 19–20

bursitis, xiv, 4, 12, 35

cables, 128; Bent Over Cable Lateral, 130, 133; Seated Cable Row, 130, 135; Seated One-Arm Cross Cable Lateral, 130, 134; Standing Cable External Rotation, 130, 132; Standing Cable Lateral, 130, 134–35

calcific tendinitis, 16–17, 35

capsules, 4, 5

CAT scan. *See* CT scan

cavitations, 29

Chest Dip, 113–15

Chest Fly, 116

Chest Stretch: Arm Across Chest Stretch, 68–69, *69*; Doorway Chest Stretch, 71; as harmful for shoulder problems, 115

chin: retractions, 106–7; tucks, 106

chiropractors, 25, 26, 28

chronic tear, 20

circulatory problems, 47

clavicle, 2

cold allergies, 47

collarbone. *See* clavicle

computer monitor screen, and sitting posture, 95

construction job exercises, 147–48

construction workers, 147–48, *148*

cortisone shots, 42–43

critical zone, 20

CT scan: MRI compared to, 34; overview, 32

dead-arm syndrome, xiv

desk job exercises, 148–49

diabetes, 47

diagnostic tests, 30–35. *See also specific tests*

diagnostic ultrasound, 34–35

diet therapy, 50–52

doctor in osteopathic medicine (DO), 30. *See also* osteopaths

doctors: treatment and, 25–35. *See also specific doctors*

Doorway Chest Stretch, 71

Dumbbell Press, 135, 136–37, *137*

dumbbells, 128; Dumbbell Bench Press, 119; Dumbbell Press, 135, 136–37, *137*; Front Dumbbell Raise, 135–36; Seated Bent Over Dumbbell Raise, 130, 131, *132*

eating. *See* diet therapy

Empty-Can Fly, 120

exercises: General Adaptation Syndrome, 124; injuries and, xvi; isotonic, 72; overdoing, 49–50; overview, xv–xvi, 59, 64, 85; patience and, 48–49; reps, sets and rest, 59, 60–63; ROM, 48, 49, 64–71; rotator cuff training, 129, 154n3; stretching, 63–64; warm-up, 59, 60, 114. *See also* harmful exercises, for shoulder problems; posture exercises; ROM exercises; strengthening exercises; workouts; *specific exercise topics*

extension, 3

external rotation, 3, 121; Isometric External Rotation, 73; Side Lying External Rotation, 74–76, *75*, *76*

Face Pull, 135, 138–39, *139*, *140*

falling, 18

faulty posture: flat back, 99–100; kyphotic-lordotic back, 101–2; layer syndrome, 104; lower cross body syndrome, 103, 104; swayback, 99–101; Upper Crossed Syndrome, 90, 91, 104. *See also* posture exercises

fixes. *See* exercises; treatment

flat back posture, 99–100

flexion, 3

football exercises, 143–44

Forward Alphabet in Sitting, 82

forward head posture: exercises, 105–7; overview, 89–91; Upper Crossed Syndrome and, 90, 91

Front Dumbbell Raise, 135–36

frozen shoulder, xiv; overview, 14–16, 35

full thickness tear, 20, 152n2

General Adaptation Syndrome, 124

general practitioner, 29

G/H joint. *See* glenohumeral joint

Gironda, Vince, 119

glenohumeral (G/H) joint, 3

glenoid fossa, 2

golf exercises, 142

greater tubercle, 2, 22

guillotine press, 119. *See also* Neck Bench Press

gymnastic exercises, 146–47

handedness, and posture, 101–2

harmful exercises, for shoulder problems: Barbell Behind-The-Neck Press, 116–17; Chest Dip, 113–15; Chest Fly, 116; Chest Stretch, 115; Dumbbell Bench Press, 119; Lat Pull-Down Behind Neck, 118–19; Neck Bench Press, 119–20; overview, 112–13; Push-Ups, 121–22; Supraspinatus Fly, 120–21; Upright Row, 117–18

health, and posture, 87

health-care practitioners, 36. *See also* doctors; *specific health practitioners*

heat: ice compared to, 44–45; using, 45

herbal remedies, 52

hockey exercises, 146

horizontal adduction, 68

humerus, 2

hydroxyapatite, 16

hypertension, 47

ice: heat compared to, 44–45; overview, 43–44, *44*; using, 45–48

impingement syndrome, 152n4; overview, 11, 21–23, 152n3; primary and secondary types, 21–23, 35

inferential current, 43, *43*

inflammation, 44–45

infraspinatus muscle, 5, *5*, 6

injuries: acute, 47; biomechanical, 18; examples, xi–xii, 37; exercises and, xvi; nontraumatic, 37–38; overview, xiii, 11; secondary hypoxic, 45; separated shoulder, 4; shoulder movement and, xvi, 1–2; traumatic, 18; workouts and, 112. *See also* rotator cuff injuries; shoulder problems; *specific injuries*

insertions, 2

internal rotation, 3, 121

intratendinous tears, 19, 20

isometric exercises, 72; Isometric External Rotation, 73; Isometric Shoulder Abduction, 73–74, *74*; Isometric Shoulder Flexion, 73

isotonic exercises, 72

itis, 11–12

Janda, Vladimir, 90, 103

Jobe, Frank, 120

joints: acromioclavicular, 3, 4, 113; glenohumeral, 3; overview, 2–4; scapulothoracic, 3, 4; shoulder, 3; sternoclavicular, 3, 4 kyphotic-lordotic back, 101–2

Latissimus Dorsi (lats), 9
Latissimus Dorsi Stretch, 70–71
Lat Pull-Down Behind Neck, 118–19
lats muscles. *See* Latissimus Dorsi
layer syndrome, 104
left-handedness posture, 103
lifting, 17
ligaments, 4
LOS. *See* lower cross body syndrome
lower body, and posture, 97–98
lower cross body syndrome (LOS), 103,
    104
lower trapezius, 7
lumbar spine, 99

magnetic resonant imaging (MRI), *33*;
    CT scan compared to, 34; overview,
    30–32; X-ray compared to, 32–34
manipulations, 28–29
mattresses, and posture, 107–8
medical doctor (MD), 30
medications, 41. *See also specific*
    medications
mobilizations, 28
movement. *See* range of motion;
    shoulder movement
MRI. *See* magnetic resonant imaging
muscles: diet therapy and, 50; guarding
    and spasms, 48; imbalances, 18;
    infraspinatus, 5, *5*, 6; Latissimus
    Dorsi, 9; pectoralis, 9; rotator cuff,
    xv, *5*, 5–7, 9; scapular stabilizing,
    7–9; strengthening in prevention
    exercises, 123–25; subscapularis, 5, *5*,
    6; supporting, xiv; supraspinatus, 5, *5*,
    6; teres minor, 5, *5*, 6; trapezius, 7–8;
    weakened, 98. *See also specific muscles*
muscle spasms, 48; posture and, 94

Neck Bench Press, 119–20
Neer, Charles, 152n3
nontraumatic injuries, 37–38

One Arm Bent Row, 130, 134
origins, 2
ortho-out clinic, 27
orthopedics, 27
orthopedic surgeons, 19, 29, 30
osteopaths, 25–26, *26*, 30
osteopathy, 25–26, 28

pain, 12–13; posture and, 92–93;
    treatment for, xiii. *See also* shoulder
    pain
partial thickness tear, 19
pecs. *See* pectoralis muscles
pectoralis major, 9
pectoralis minor, 8
pectoralis muscles, 9
Pelvic Tilt, 101
pelvis, anteriorly tipped, 102
Pendulum Exercises, 66–67
physiatrist, 29–30
physical therapy, 27–28, 152n4
physiotherapists (PTs), 25, *27*, 27–28, 30
physiotherapy. *See* physical therapy
Pilates: overview and principles, 54–57;
    reformer, 54–55, *55*
Pilates, Joseph, 54
Plank exercise, 101
posterior chain, 97
posture: abdominal crunches and, 105;
    forward head, 89–91, 105–7; good,
    87–88, 91, 98–99; handedness and,
    101–3; health and, 87; ideal, 92, 99;
    leaning forward, 97; left-handedness
    and, 103; lower body, 97–98;
    mattresses, sleeping and, 107–8;
    muscle spasms and, 94; overview,
    xvi, 87, 110; pain and, 92–93; poor,
    17, 19, 88–89, 91–92; power and,
    98–99; proper positioning, 92–93;
    right-handedness and, 102–3;
    shoulder pain and, 38; standing, 97;
    thoracic outlet syndrome and, 91–
    92; tips, 110. *See also* faulty posture;
    sitting posture

posture bra, 109
posture braces, 109
posture exercises: for forward head, 105–7; overview, 104–5; Pelvic Tilt, 101; Plank, 101
power, and posture, 98–99
preventative treatment, xiii
prevention exercises: overview, 123; strengthening muscles, 123–25. *See also* super shoulder workouts
primary care physician, 29
primary impingement syndrome, 21–23, 35
PTs. *See* physiotherapists
Push-Ups: as harmful for shoulder problems, 121–22; Shoulder Blade, 78

range of motion (ROM), 13. *See also* ROM exercises; shoulder ROM
rehabilitation doctor. *See* physiatrist
repetitions. *See* reps
repetitive faulty movements, 18
reps: concentric phase, 61; eccentric phase, 61; overview, 60–61; sets, rest and, 59, 60–63
Reynaud's phenomenon, 47
rhomboid major, 7
rhomboid minor, 7
rhomboids, 7
rib cage, 25, 151n2
right-handedness posture, 102–3
ROM. *See* range of motion
ROM exercises: Arm Across Chest Stretch, 68–69, *69*; Doorway Chest Stretch, 71; Latissimus Dorsi Stretch, 70–71; overview, 48, *49*, 64–65; Pendulum Exercises, 66–67; Standing Front Wall Walking, 67, *67*; Standing Side Wall Walking, 68, *68*; Supine Stick Flexion, *65*, 65–66, *66*; Thoracic Spine Extension Mobility Exercise, 69–70, *70*

rotator cuff, *12*; muscles, xv, *5*, 5–7, 9; overview, xiv, xv; routines, 83–85; training exercises, 129, 154n3; weakness as shoulder problem cause, xv
rotator cuff injuries, 3, *12*; causes, 17–19; signs and symptoms, 16–17; as swimmer's shoulder, 144; tears, 19–20, 36

scaption, 130–31; Scaption with a Shrug, 130–31
scapula, 2. *See also* shoulder blades
scapular dyskinesis, 22
scapular plane elevation, 130. *See also* scaption
scapular stabilizing muscles, 7–9
scapulothoracic (S/T) joint, 3, 4
sciatica (shin splints), 11
S/C joint. *See* sternoclavicular joint
seated exercises: Seated Bent Over Dumbbell Raise, 130, 131, *132*; Seated Cable Row, 130, 135; Seated One-Arm Cross Cable Lateral, 130, 134
secondary hypoxic injury, 45
secondary impingement syndrome, 21–23, 35
separated shoulder, 4
serratus anterior, 7, 8
sets: overview, 61–62; reps, rest and, 59, 60–63
shin splints, 11
shoulder: overview, xiii, 1–2, 10. *See also specific topics*
shoulder blades, 2
shoulder blades exercise, 107; Shoulder Blade Push-Up, 78
shoulder fixes. *See* exercises; treatment
shoulder impingement syndrome, 11. *See also* impingement syndrome
shoulder joint, 3. *See also* glenohumeral joint

shoulder movement: injuries and, xvi, 1–2; overview, xiii, 1–2; repetitive faulty, 18. *See also* shoulder ROM

shoulder pain: examples, xi–xii; moving on and keeping at bay, 48–50; from nontraumatic injuries, 25; overview, xii–xv, 11, 57; posture and, 38; rib cage and, 25, 151n2; as signal, 39–41. *See also specific shoulder pain topics*

shoulder problems: causes, xiv, xv; results, xiv. *See also* harmful exercises, for shoulder problems; injuries; *specific problems*

Shoulder Raise in Sitting, 81, *81*

shoulder ROM, xiii;13. *See also* ROM exercises; shoulder movement

shoulder trouble. *See* shoulder problems

side lying exercises: Side Lying Alphabet, 78; Side Lying Arm Straight Up, 76–77, *77*; Side Lying External Rotation, 74–76, *75, 76*; Side Lying Lateral Raise, 135, 137–38

sitting exercises: Alphabet with Your Arm at Side in Sitting, 82–83; Arm to Your Side in Sitting, 82; desk job, 148–49; Forward Alphabet in Sitting, 82; Shoulder Raise in Sitting, 81, *81*

sitting posture, 19, 23, 89; checklist for optimum, 96; computer monitor screen and, 95; dynamic sitting, 94–95; improper, *96*; proper, *93*

sleep: posture and, 107–8; tendinitis and, 24–25

softball exercises, 141–42

spine: ideal, 87; lumbar, 99

sports exercises: baseball and softball, 141–42; basketball, 145–46; football, 143–44; golf, 142; gymnastics, 146–47; hockey, 146; overview, 140–41; swimming, 144–45; tennis, 142–43

stabilizing muscles. *See* scapular stabilizing muscles

standing exercises: Standing Cable External Rotation, 130, 132; Standing Cable Lateral, 130, 134–35; Standing Front Wall Walking, 67, *67*; Standing Lateral Raise, 135, 138; Standing Side Wall Walking, 68, *68*

standing posture, 97

static stretching, 63–64

sternoclavicular (S/C) joint, 3, 4

S/T joint. *See* scapulothoracic joint

stratification syndrome, 104

strengthening exercises: Airplane Exercise, 78–79, *79*; Alphabet with Your Arm at Side in Sitting, 82–83; Arm to Your Side in Sitting, 82; Forward Alphabet in Sitting, 82; Isometric External Rotation, 73; Isometric Shoulder Abduction, 73–74, *74*; Isometric Shoulder Flexion, 73; overview, 48, 49, 71–72; Shoulder Blade Push-Up, 78; Shoulder Raise in Sitting, 81, *81*; Side Lying Alphabet, 78; Side Lying Arm Straight Up, 76–77, *77*; Side Lying External Rotation, 74–76, *75, 76*; Superman Exercise, 80, *80, 81*

stress, 23–24

stretching, 63–64; Latissimus Dorsi Stretch, 70–71. *See also* Chest Stretch

subacromial bursa, 22

subacromial space, 22

subacromial syndrome, 152n3. *See also* impingement syndrome

subscapularis muscle, 5, *5*, 6

Superman Exercise, 80, *80, 81*

super shoulder workouts: beginning weights, 127–29; construction job, 147–48; desk job, 148–49; duration of, 129; frequency and weight amount, 126–27; overview, 125–29. *See also* advanced exercises;

beginner exercises; prevention exercises; sports exercises
supination, 9
Supine Stick Flexion, *65*, 65–66, *66*
supplements, 52
supporting muscles, xiv
Supraspinatus Fly, 120–21
supraspinatus muscle, 5, *5*, 6
supraspinatus tendon, 20
surgeons, orthopedic, 19, 29, 30
surgery, 30, 152n2
surgical debridement, 20
surgical decompression, arthroscopic, 152n4
swayback, 99–101
swimmer's friction shoulder, 144
swimmer's shoulder, 11, 144
swimming exercises, 144–45

tears, rotator cuff, 19–20, 36, 152n2
tendinitis, xiv; calcific, 16–17, 35; causes, 13–14; overview, 11–12, *12*, 35; signs and symptoms, 16–17; sleep and, 24–25
tendinosis, 14
tendonitis. *See* tendinitis
tendons: diet therapy and, 50–51; overview, 4; supraspinatus, 20
tennis exercises, 142–43
Teres Major, 9
teres minor muscle, 5, *5*, 6
thoracic outlet syndrome (TOC), 91–92
Thoracic Spine Extension Mobility Exercise, 69–70, *70*
thrower's shoulder, 11

TOC. *See* thoracic outlet syndrome
traction, 106
trapezius ("trap") muscle, 7–8
traumatic injuries, 18
treatment: doctors and, 25–35; overview, xiii, xv, 13, 150; preventative, xiii; of rotator cuff muscles, xv; for weakness and pain, xiii. *See also* exercises; *specific treatment topics*

ultrasound, 34–35
Upper Crossed Syndrome, 104; forward head posture and, 90, 91
Upright Row, 117–18

warm-up, 59, 60, 114
weight training: beginning weights, 127–29; dumbbells, barbells and cables overview, 128; frequency and amount, 126–27; General Adaptation Syndrome, 124. *See also* super shoulder workouts; *specific weight training exercises*
weight training repetitions. *See* reps
workouts: injuries and, 112; overview, 111–12. *See also* exercises; super shoulder workouts
wounds, 47

X-rays: arthrograms using, 35; MRIs compared to, 32–34; overview, *31*, 31–32

yoga, 53–54